The Only
EKG
BOOK

You'll Ever Need

SEVENTH EDITION

MALCOLM S. THALER, M.D.

 Wolters Kluwer | Lippincott Williams & Wilkins
Health
Philadelphia · Baltimore · New York · London
Buenos Aires · Hong Kong · Sydney · Tokyo

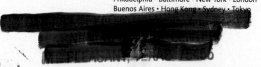

Senior Acquisitions Editor: Sonya Seigafuse
Senior Product Manager: Kerry Barrett
Production Manager: Bridgett Dougherty
Senior Manufacturing Manager: Benjamin Rivera
Senior Marketing Manager: Kimberly Schonberger
Design Coordinator: Terry Mallon
Production Service: SPi Global

Printed in China

Library of Congress Cataloging-in-Publication Data
Thaler, Malcolm S.
  The only EKG book you'll ever need / Malcolm S. Thaler. — 7th ed.
      p. ; cm.
  Includes index.
  ISBN 978-1-4511-1905-3
  I. Title.
  [DNLM: 1. Electrocardiography. 2. Heart Diseases—diagnosis. WG 140]
  616.1′207547—dc23

                                                                                    2011041429

Care has been taken to confirm the accuracy of the information presented and to describe generally accepted practices. However, the authors, editors, and publisher are not responsible for errors or omissions or for any consequences from application of the information in this book and make no warranty, expressed or implied, with respect to the currency, completeness, or accuracy of the contents of the publication. Application of the information in a particular situation remains the professional responsibility of the practitioner.

The authors, editors, and publisher have exerted every effort to ensure that drug selection and dosage set forth in this text are in accordance with current recommendations and practice at the time of publication. However, in view of ongoing research, changes in government regulations, and the constant flow of information relating to drug therapy and drug reactions, the reader is urged to check the package insert for each drug for any change in indications and dosage and for added warnings and precautions. This is particularly important when the recommended agent is a new or infrequently employed drug.

Some drugs and medical devices presented in the publication have Food and Drug Administration (FDA) clearance for limited use in restricted research settings. It is the responsibility of the health care provider to ascertain the FDA status of each drug or device planned for use in their clinical practice.

To purchase additional copies of this book, call our customer service department at (800) 638-3030 or fax orders to (301) 223-2320. International customers should call (301) 223-2300.

Visit Lippincott Williams & Wilkins on the Internet: at LWW.com. Lippincott Williams & Wilkins customer service representatives are available from 8:30 am to 6 pm, EST.

10 9 8 7 6 5 4 3

RRS1401

Dedication

To Nancy, Ali, and Jon—of course

Preface

New content! New cases! New color! New clinical pearls! Yet even as we keep adding, changing, and improving, the fundamentals remain. It's been about 25 years since the first edition of this little book, and we have remained resolute to the principles outlined in that very first preface:

This book is about learning. It's about keeping simple things simple and complicated things clear, concise and, yes, simple, too. It's about getting from here to there without scaring you to death, boring you to tears, or intimidating your socks off. It's about turning ignorance into knowledge, knowledge into wisdom, and all with a bit of fun.

We must be doing something right, because each year *The Only EKG Book You Will Ever Need* becomes more popular, more widely translated, and adopted and used in more medical and other professional schools. This edition offers a host of revisions and refinements:

A whole new palette of colors to make the models, illustrations, and tracings clearer than ever

New clinical cases to expand on one of the most important distinctions of the book: to put everything into its proper clinical context (you are put right into the middle of real-life clinical situations) and to make the information *usable*

Expanded sections on subjects where new developments have made deeper understanding possible, including atrial fibrillation, long QT syndrome, apical ballooning syndrome, and others

Greater clarity where it is called for, new tracings where they help illuminate the points we are trying to make, and—wherever possible—shortening and simplifying

As ever, hats off to Glenn Harper, M.D., the world's greatest cardiologist, whose help was invaluable in ensuring the text is up-to-date, clear, and accurate. And remove two more hats for Kerry Barrett and Sonya Seigafuse, who continue to lead the Lippincott Williams & Wilkins team that—year after year, edition after edition—produces the best-looking, most readable EKG book that one could hope for.

To those of you who are picking up this book for the first time and for those of you who are making a return visit, I hope *The Only EKG Book You Will Ever Need* will provide you with everything *you* need to read EKGs quickly and accurately.

Malcolm Thaler, M.D.

Contents

[1]Practice, practice, practice!

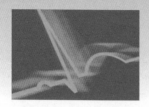

Getting Started

In this chapter you will learn:

1 | not a thing, but don't worry. There is plenty to come. Here is your
chance to turn a few pages and get yourself settled and ready to roll.
Relax. Pour some tea. Begin.

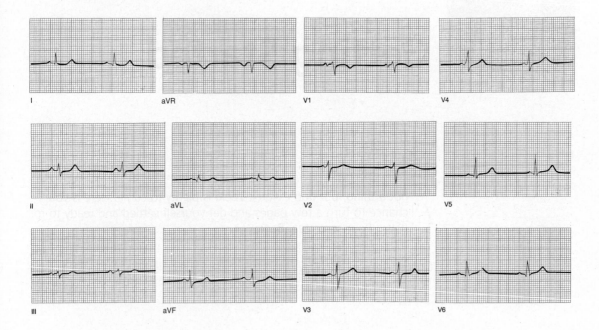

I	aVR	V1	V4
II	aVL	V2	V5
III	aVF	V3	V6

On the opposite page is a normal electrocardiogram, or EKG. By the time you have finished this book—and it won't take very much time at all—you will be able to recognize a normal EKG almost instantly. Perhaps even more importantly, you will have learned to spot all of the common abnormalities that can occur on an EKG, and you will be good at it!

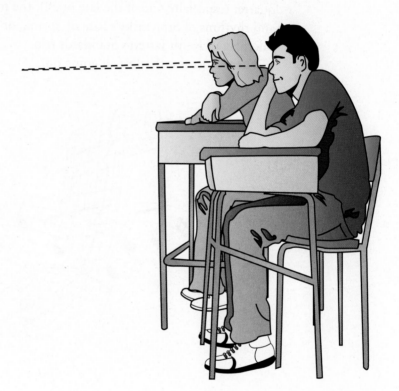

Some people have compared learning to read EKGs with learning to read music. In both instances, one is faced with a completely new notational system not rooted in conventional language and full of unfamiliar shapes and symbols.

But there really is no comparison. The simple lub-dub of the heart cannot approach the subtle complexity of a Beethoven string quartet (especially one of the late ones!), the multiplying tonalities and rhythms of Stravinsky's Rite of Spring, or the extraordinary jazz interplay of Keith Jarrett's Standards trio.

There's just not that much going on.

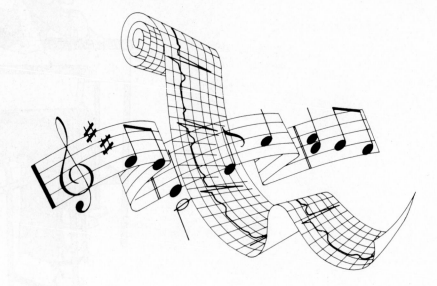

The EKG is a tool of remarkable clinical power, remarkable both for the ease with which it can be mastered and for the extraordinary range of situations in which it can provide helpful and even critical information. One glance at an EKG can diagnose an evolving myocardial infarction, identify a potentially life-threatening arrhythmia, pinpoint the chronic effects of sustained hypertension or the acute effects of a massive pulmonary embolus, or simply provide a measure of reassurance to someone who wants to begin an exercise program.

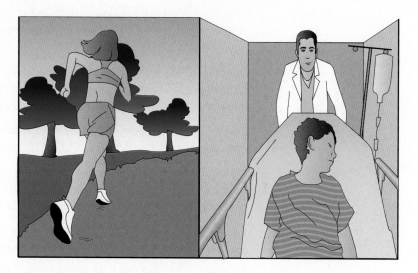

Remember, however, that the EKG is only a tool and, like any tool, is only as capable as its user. Put a chisel in my hand and you are unlikely to get Michelangelo's *David*.

The nine chapters of this book will take you on an electrifying voyage from ignorance to dazzling competence. You will amaze your friends (and, more importantly, yourself). The road map you will follow looks like this:

Chapter 1: You will learn about the electrical events that generate the different waves on the EKG, and—armed with this knowledge—you will be able to recognize and understand the normal 12-lead EKG.

Chapter 2: You will see how simple and predictable alterations in certain waves permit the diagnosis of enlargement and hypertrophy of the atria and ventricles.

Chapter 3: You will become familiar with the most common disturbances in cardiac rhythm and will learn why some are life threatening while others are merely nuisances.

Chapter 4: You will learn to identify interruptions in the normal pathways of cardiac conduction and will be introduced to pacemakers.

Chapter 5: As a complement to Chapter 4, you will learn what happens when the electrical current bypasses the usual channels of conduction and arrives more quickly at its destination.

Chapter 6: You will learn to diagnose ischemic heart disease: myocardial infarctions (heart attacks) and angina (ischemic heart pain).

Chapter 7: You will see how various noncardiac phenomena can alter the EKG.

Chapter 8: You will put all your newfound knowledge together into a simple 11-step method for reading all EKGs.

Chapter 9: A few practice strips will let you test your knowledge and revel in your astonishing intellectual growth.

The whole process is straightforward and should not be the least bit intimidating. Intricacies of thought and great leaps of creative logic are not required.

This is not the time for deep thinking.

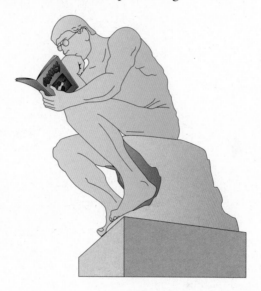

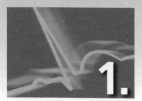

1. The Basics

In this chapter you will learn:

1 | how the electrical current in the heart is generated

2 | how this current is propagated through the four chambers of the heart

3 | that the movement of electricity through the heart produces predictable wave patterns on the EKG

4 | how the EKG machine detects and records these waves

5 | that the EKG looks at the heart from 12 different perspectives

6 | that you are now able to recognize and *understand* all the lines and waves on the 12-lead EKG.

Electricity and the Heart

Electricity, an innate biologic electricity, is what makes the heart go. The EKG is nothing more than a recording of the heart's electrical activity, and it is through perturbations in the normal electrical patterns that we are able to diagnose many different cardiac disorders.

All You Need to Know About Cellular Electrophysiology in Two Pages

Cardiac cells, in their resting state, are electrically polarized; that is, their insides are negatively charged with respect to their outsides. This electrical polarity is maintained by membrane pumps that ensure the appropriate distribution of ions (primarily potassium, sodium, chloride, and calcium) necessary to keep the insides of these cells relatively electronegative. These ions pass into and out of the cell through special ion channels in the cell membrane.

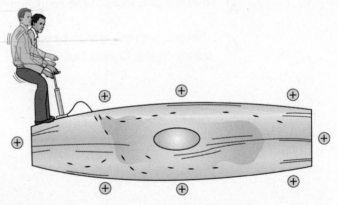

The resting cardiac cell maintains its electrical polarity by means of a membrane pump. This pump requires a constant supply of energy, and the gentleman above, were he real rather than a visual metaphor, would soon be flat on his back.

Cardiac cells can lose their internal negativity in a process called *depolarization*. **Depolarization is the fundamental electrical event of the heart.** In some cells, known as pacemaker cells, it occurs spontaneously. In others, it is initiated by the arrival of an electrical impulse that causes positively charged ions to cross the cell membrane.

Depolarization is propagated from cell to cell, producing a wave of depolarization that can be transmitted across the entire heart. This wave of depolarization represents a flow of electricity, an electrical current, that can be detected by electrodes placed on the surface of the body.

After depolarization is complete, the cardiac cells restore their resting polarity through a process called *repolarization*. Repolarization is accomplished by the membrane pumps, which reverse the flow of ions. This process can also be detected by recording electrodes.

All of the different waves that we see on an EKG are manifestations of these two processes: depolarization and repolarization.

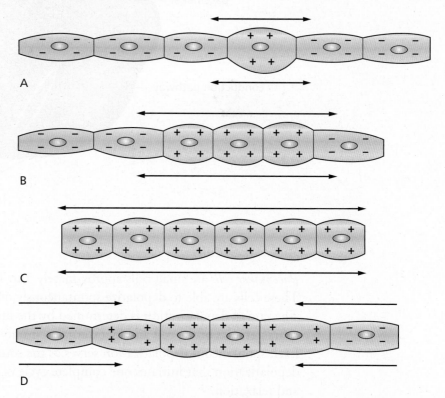

In *A*, a single cell has depolarized. A wave of depolarization then propagates from cell to cell (*B*) until all are depolarized (*C*). Repolarization (*D*) then restores each cell's resting polarity.

The Cells of the Heart

From the standpoint of the electrocardiographer, the heart consists of three types of cells:

- *Pacemaker cells*—under normal circumstances, the electrical power source of the heart

- *Electrical conducting cells*—the hard wiring of the heart

- *Myocardial cells*—the contractile machinery of the heart.

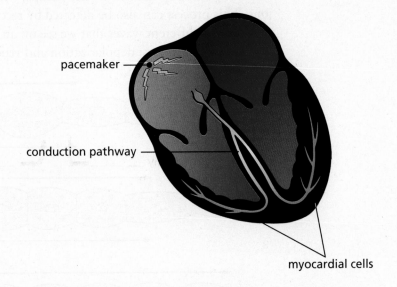

Pacemaker Cells

Pacemaker cells are small cells approximately 5 to 10 μm long. These cells are able to depolarize spontaneously over and over again. The rate of depolarization is determined by the innate electrical characteristics of the cell and by external neurohormonal input. Each spontaneous depolarization serves as the source of a wave of depolarization that initiates one complete cycle of cardiac contraction and relaxation.

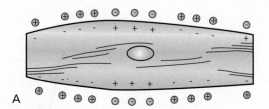

A pacemaker cell depolarizing spontaneously.

If we record one electrical cycle of depolarization and repolarization from a single cell, we get an electrical tracing called an **action potential.** With each spontaneous depolarization, a new action potential is generated, which in turn stimulates neighboring cells to depolarize and generate their own action potential, and so on and on, until the entire heart has been depolarized.

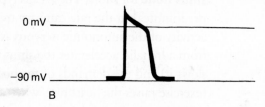

A typical action potential.

The action potential of a cardiac pacemaker cell looks a little different from the generic action potential shown here. A pacemaker cell does *not* have a true resting potential. Its electrical charge drops to a minimal negative potential, which it maintains for just a moment (it does not rest there), and then rises gradually until it reaches the threshold for the sudden depolarization that is an action potential. These events are illustrated on the following tracing.

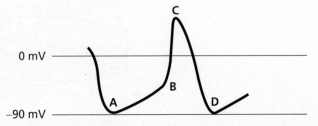

0 mV

−90 mV

The electrical depolarization–repolarization cycle of a cardiac pacemaker cell. Point *A* is the minimal negative potential. The gentle rising slope between points *A* and *B* represents a slow, gradual depolarization. At point *B*, the threshold is crossed and the cell dramatically depolarizes (as seen between points B and C); that is, an action potential is produced. The downslope between points *C* and *D* represents repolarization. This cycle will repeat over and over for, let us hope, many, many years.

The dominant pacemaker cells in the heart are located high up in the right atrium. This group of cells is called the **sinoatrial (SA) node,** or **sinus node** for short. These cells typically fire at a rate of 60 to 100 times per minute, but the rate can vary tremendously depending upon the activity of the autonomic nervous system (*e.g.*, sympathetic stimulation from adrenalin accelerates the sinus node, whereas vagal stimulation slows it) and the demands of the body for increased cardiac output (exercise raises the heart rate, whereas a restful afternoon nap lowers it).

Pacemaker cells are really good at what they do. They will continue firing in a donor heart even after it has been harvested for transplant and before it has been connected to the new recipient.

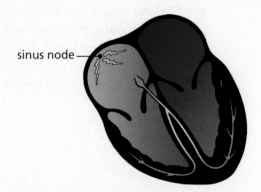

sinus node

In a resting individual, the sinus node typically fires 60 to 100 times per minute, producing a regular series of action potentials, each of which initiates a wave of depolarization that will spread through the heart.

Actually, *every* cell in the heart has the ability to behave like a pace-maker cell. This so-called *automatic ability* is normally suppressed unless the dominant cells of the sinus node fail or if something in the internal or external environment of a cell (sympathetic stimulation, cardiac disease, *etc.*) stimulates its automatic behavior. This topic assumes greater importance later on and is discussed under *Ectopic Rhythms* in Chapter 3.

Electrical Conducting Cells

Electrical conducting cells are long, thin cells. Like the wires of an electrical circuit, these cells carry current rapidly and efficiently to distant regions of the heart. The electrical conducting cells of the ventricles form distinct electrical pathways. The ventricular conducting fibers comprise the *Purkinje system*.

The conducting pathways in the atria have more anatomic variability; prominent among these are fibers at the top of the intra-atrial septum in a region called Bachman's bundle that allow for rapid activation of the left atrium from the right.

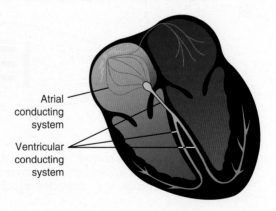

Atrial conducting system

Ventricular conducting system

The hard wiring of the heart.

Myocardial Cells

The *myocardial cells* constitute by far the largest part of the heart tissue. They are responsible for the heavy labor of repeatedly contracting and relaxing, thereby delivering blood to the rest of the body. These cells are about 50 to 100 μm in length and contain an abundance of the contractile proteins actin and myosin.

When a wave of depolarization reaches a myocardial cell, calcium is released within the cell, causing the cell to contract. This process, in which calcium plays the key intermediary role, is called *excitation–contraction coupling.*

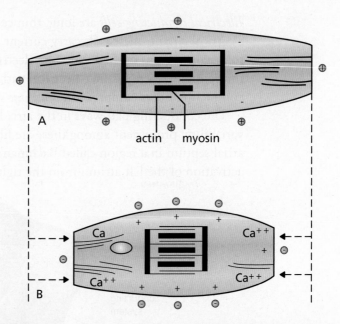

Depolarization causes calcium to be released within a myocardial cell. This influx of calcium allows actin and myosin, the contractile proteins, to interact, causing the cell to contract. (*A*) A resting myocardial cell. (*B*) A depolarized, contracted myocardial cell.

Myocardial cells can transmit an electrical current just like electrical conducting cells, but they do so far less efficiently. Thus, a wave of depolarization, upon reaching the myocardial cells, will spread slowly across the entire myocardium.

Time and Voltage

The waves that appear on an EKG primarily reflect the electrical activity of the *myocardial cells,* which compose the vast bulk of the heart. Pacemaker activity and transmission by the conducting system are generally not seen on the EKG; these events simply do not generate sufficient voltage to be recorded by surface electrodes.

The waves produced by myocardial depolarization and repolarization are recorded on EKG paper and, like any simple wave, have three chief characteristics:

1. *Duration,* measured in fractions of a second

2. *Amplitude,* measured in millivolts (mV)

3. *Configuration,* a more subjective criterion referring to the shape and appearance of a wave.

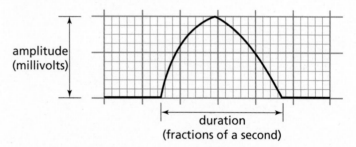

A typical wave that might be seen on any EKG. It is two large squares (or 10 small squares) in amplitude, three large squares (or 15 small squares) in duration, and slightly asymmetric in configuration.

EKG Paper

EKG paper is a long, continuous roll of graph paper, usually pink (but any color will do), with light and dark lines running vertically and horizontally. The light lines circumscribe small squares of 1 × 1 mm; the dark lines delineate large squares of 5 × 5 mm.

The horizontal axis measures time. The distance across one small square represents 0.04 seconds. The distance across one large square is five times greater, or 0.2 seconds.

The vertical axis measures voltage. The distance along one small square represents 0.1 mV, and along one large square, 0.5 mV.

You will need to memorize these numbers at some point, so you might as well do it now.

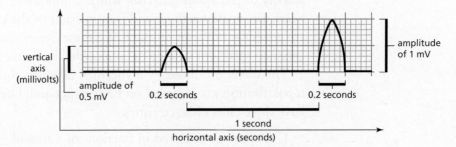

Both waves are one large square in duration (0.2 seconds), but the second wave is twice the voltage of the first (1 mV compared with 0.5 mV). The flat segment connecting the two waves is five large squares (5 × 0.2 seconds = 1 second) in duration.

P Waves, QRS Complexes, T Waves, and Some Straight Lines

Let's follow one cycle of cardiac contraction (systole) and relaxation (diastole), focusing on the electrical events that produce the basic waves and lines of the standard EKG.

Atrial Depolarization

The sinus node fires spontaneously (an event not visible on the EKG), and a wave of depolarization begins to spread outward into the atrial myocardium, much as if a pebble were dropped into a calm lake. Depolarization of the atrial myocardial cells results in atrial contraction.

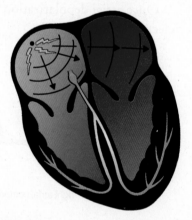

Each cycle of normal cardiac contraction and relaxation begins when the sinus node depolarizes spontaneously. The wave of depolarization then propagates through both atria, causing them to contract.

During atrial depolarization and contraction, electrodes placed on the surface of the body record a small burst of electrical activity lasting a fraction of a second. This is the *P wave*. It is a recording of the spread of depolarization through the atrial myocardium from start to finish.

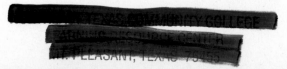
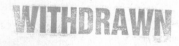

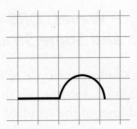

The EKG records a small deflection, the P wave.

Because the sinus node is located in the right atrium, the right atrium begins to depolarize before the left atrium and finishes earlier as well. Therefore, the first part of the P wave predominantly represents right atrial depolarization, and the second part left atrial depolarization.

Once atrial depolarization is complete, the EKG again becomes electrically silent.

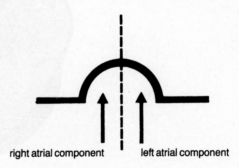

right atrial component   left atrial component

The components of the P wave.

A Pause Separates Conduction From the Atria to the Ventricles

In healthy hearts, there is an electrical gate at the junction of the atria and the ventricles. The wave of depolarization, having completed its journey through the atria, is prevented from communicating with the ventricles by the heart valves that separate the atria and ventricles. Electrical conduction must be funneled along the interventricular septum, the wall that separates the right and left ventricles. Here, a structure called the *atrioventricular (AV) node* slows conduction to a crawl. This pause lasts only a fraction of a second.

This physiologic delay in conduction is essential to allow the atria to finish contracting before the ventricles begin to contract. This clever electrical wiring of the heart permits the atria to empty their volume of blood completely into the ventricles before the ventricles contract.

Like the sinus node, the AV node is also under the influence of the autonomic nervous system. Vagal stimulation slows the current even further, whereas sympathetic stimulation accelerates the current.

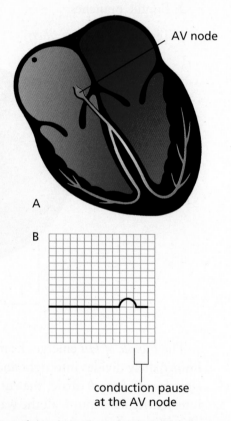

(A) The wave of depolarization is briefly held up at the AV node. (B) During this pause, the EKG falls silent; there is no detectable electrical activity.

Ventricular Depolarization

After about one-tenth of a second, the depolarizing wave escapes the AV node and is swept rapidly down the ventricles along specialized electrical conducting cells.

This ventricular conducting system has a complex anatomy but essentially consists of three parts:

1. Bundle of His

2. Bundle branches

3. Terminal *Purkinje fibers.*

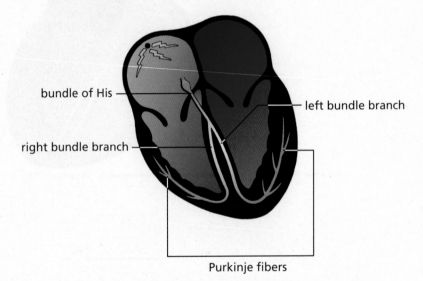

Purkinje fibers

The *bundle of His* emerges from the AV node and almost immediately divides into right and left bundle branches. The *right bundle branch* carries the current down the right side of the interventricular septum all the way to the apex of the right ventricle. The *left bundle branch* is more complicated. It divides into three major fascicles:

1. *Septal fascicle,* which depolarizes the interventricular septum (the wall of muscle separating the right and left ventricles) in a left-to-right direction

2. *Anterior fascicle,* which runs along the anterior wall of the left ventricle

3. *Posterior fascicle*, which sweeps over the posterior wall of the left ventricle.

The right bundle branch and the left bundle branch and its fascicles terminate in countless tiny Purkinje fibers, which resemble little twigs coming off the branches of a tree. These fibers deliver the electrical current into the ventricular myocardium.

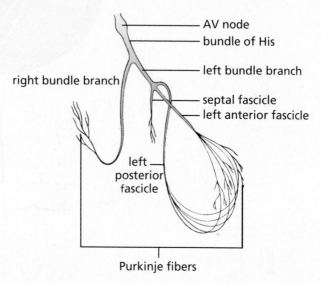

The ventricular conduction system, shown in detail. Below the bundle of His, the conduction system divides into right and left bundle branches. The right bundle branch remains intact, whereas the left divides into three separate fascicles.

Ventricular myocardial depolarization causes ventricular contraction. It is marked by a large deflection on the EKG called the *QRS complex*. The amplitude of the QRS complex is much greater than that of the atrial P wave because the ventricles have so much more muscle mass than the atria. The QRS complex is also more complicated and variable in shape, reflecting the greater intricacy of the pathway of ventricular depolarization.

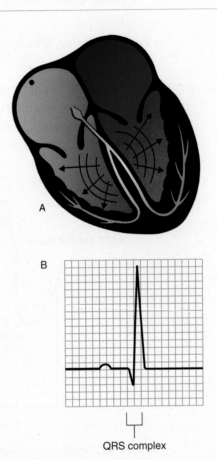

QRS complex

(*A*) Ventricular depolarization generates (*B*) a complicated waveform on the EKG called the QRS complex.

The Parts of the QRS Complex

The QRS complex consists of several distinct waves, each of which has a name. Because the precise configuration of the QRS complex can vary so greatly, a standard format for naming each component has been devised. It may seem a bit arbitrary to you right now, but it actually makes good sense.

1. If the first deflection is downward, it is called a *Q wave*.

2. The first upward deflection is called an *R wave*.

3. If there is a second upward deflection, it is called *R′* ("R-prime").

4. The first downward deflection following an upward deflection is called an *S wave*. Therefore, if the first wave of the complex is an R wave, the ensuing downward deflection is called an S wave, not a Q wave. A downward deflection can only be called a Q wave if it is the first wave of the complex. Any other downward deflection is called an S wave.

5. If the entire configuration consists solely of one downward deflection, the wave is called a *QS wave*.

Here are several of the most common QRS configurations, with each wave component named.

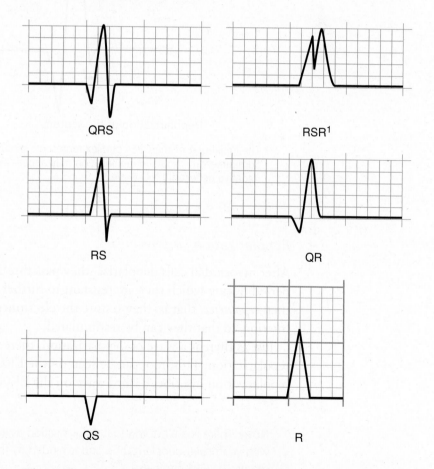

QRS

RSR¹

RS

QR

QS

R

The earliest part of the QRS complex represents depolarization of the interventricular septum by the septal fascicle of the left bundle branch. The right and left ventricles then depolarize at about the same time, but most of what we see on the EKG represents left ventricular activation because the muscle mass of the left ventricle is about three times that of the right ventricle.

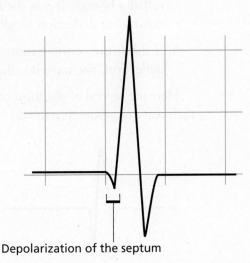

Depolarization of the septum

The initial part of the QRS complex represents septal depolarization. Sometimes, this septal depolarization may appear as a small, discrete, negative deflection, a Q wave.

Repolarization

After myocardial cells depolarize, they pass through a brief refractory period during which they are resistant to further stimulation. They then *repolarize;* that is, they restore the electronegativity of their interiors so that they can be restimulated.

Just as there is a wave of depolarization, there is also a wave of repolarization. This, too, can be seen on the EKG. Ventricular repolarization inscribes a third wave on the EKG, the *T wave.*

Note: There is a wave of atrial repolarization as well, but it coincides with ventricular depolarization and is hidden by the much more prominent QRS complex.

Ventricular repolarization is a much slower process than ventricular depolarization. Therefore, the T wave is broader than the QRS complex. Its configuration is also simpler and more rounded, like the silhouette of a gentle hill compared to the sharp, jagged, and often intricate contour of the QRS complex.

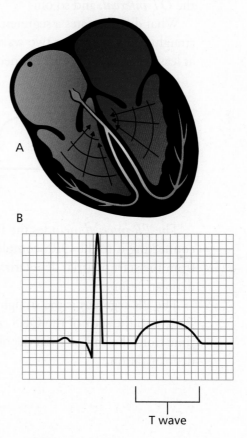

(*A*) Ventricular repolarization generates (*B*) a T wave on the EKG.

Naming the Straight Lines

The different straight lines connecting the various waves have also been given names. Thus, we speak of the *PR interval*, the *ST segment*, the *QT interval*, and so on.

What differentiates a segment from an interval? A segment is a straight line connecting two waves, whereas an interval encompasses at least one wave plus the connecting straight line.

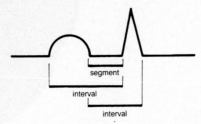

The *PR interval* includes the P wave and the straight line connecting it to the QRS complex. It therefore measures the time from the start of atrial depolarization to the start of ventricular depolarization.

The PR segment is the straight line running from the end of the P wave to the start of the QRS complex. It therefore measures the time from the end of atrial depolarization to the start of ventricular depolarization.

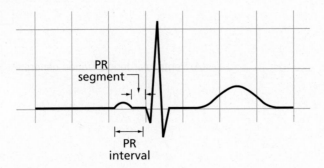

The *ST segment* is the straight line connecting the end of the QRS complex with the beginning of the T wave. It measures the time from the end of ventricular depolarization to the start of ventricular repolarization.

The *QT interval* includes the QRS complex, the ST segment, and the T wave. It therefore measures the time from the beginning of ventricular depolarization to the end of ventricular repolarization.

The term *QRS interval* is used to describe the duration of the QRS complex alone without any connecting segments. Obviously, it measures the duration of ventricular depolarization.

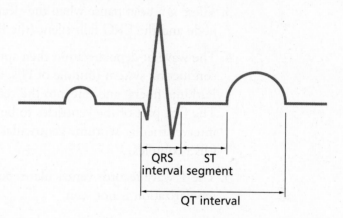

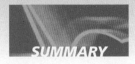

The Waves and Straight Lines of the EKG

1. Each cycle of cardiac contraction and relaxation is initiated by spontaneous depolarization of the sinus node. This event is not seen on the EKG.

2. The P wave records atrial depolarization and contraction. The first part of the P wave reflects right atrial activity; the second part reflects left atrial activity.

3. There is a brief pause when the electrical current reaches the AV node and the EKG falls silent (the PR segment).

4. The wave of depolarization then spreads along the ventricular conducting system (bundle of His, bundle branches, and Purkinje fibers) and out into the ventricular myocardium. The first part of the ventricles to be depolarized is the interventricular septum. Ventricular depolarization generates the QRS complex.

5. The T wave records ventricular repolarization. Atrial repolarization is not seen.

6. Various segments and intervals describe the time between these events:

    a. The PR interval measures the time from the start of atrial depolarization to the start of ventricular depolarization.

    b. The PR segment measures the time from the end of atrial depolarization to the start of ventricular depolarization.

    c. The ST segment records the time from the end of ventricular depolarization to the start of ventricular repolarization.

d. The QT interval measures the time from the start of ventricular depolarization to the end of ventricular repolarization.

e. The QRS interval measures the time of ventricular depolarization.

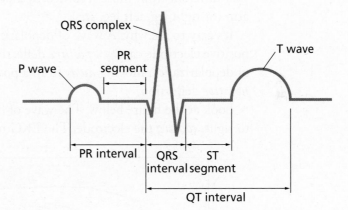

Making Waves

Electrodes can be placed anywhere on the surface of the body to record the heart's electrical activity. If we do this, we quickly discover that the waves recorded by a positive electrode on the left arm look very different from those recorded by a positive electrode on the right arm (or right leg, left leg, *etc.*).

It's easy to see why. A wave of depolarization moving *toward* a positive electrode causes a *positive* deflection on the EKG. A wave of depolarization moving *away* from a positive electrode causes a *negative* deflection.

Look at the figure below. The wave of depolarization is moving left to right, *toward* the electrode. The EKG records a positive deflection.

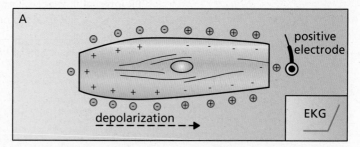

A wave of depolarization moving toward a positive electrode records a positive deflection on the EKG.

Now look at the following figure. The wave of depolarization is moving right to left, *away* from the electrode. The EKG therefore records a negative deflection.

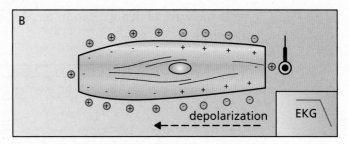

A wave of depolarization moving away from a positive electrode records a negative deflection on the EKG.

What will the EKG record if the positive electrode is placed in the middle of the cell?

Initially, as the wavefront approaches the electrode, the EKG records a positive deflection.

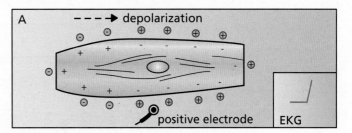

Depolarization begins, generating a positive deflection on the EKG.

Then, at the precise moment that the wave reaches the electrode, the positive and negative charges are balanced and essentially cancel each other out. The EKG recording returns to baseline.

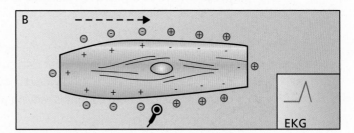

The wavefront reaches the electrode. The positive and negative charges are balanced, and the EKG returns to baseline.

As the wave of depolarization recedes, a negative deflection is inscribed.

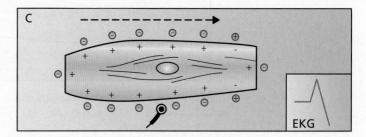

The wave of depolarization begins to recede from the electrode, generating a negative deflection.

The EKG finally returns to baseline once again when depolarization is complete.

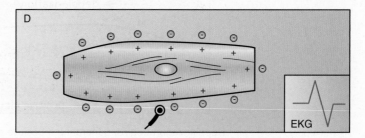

The cell is fully depolarized, and the EKG once again returns to baseline.

The final inscription of a depolarizing wave moving perpendicularly to a positive electrode is therefore a *biphasic wave*.

What would the tracing look like if the recording electrode were placed over a region of pacemaker cells sufficient to generate a detectable current? The tracing would show a downward, negative deflection, since all the current is moving away from the origin where you are recording.

The effects of repolarization on the EKG are similar to those of depolarization, except that the charges are reversed. A wave of repolarization moving *toward* a positive electrode inscribes a *negative* deflection on the EKG. A wave of repolarization moving *away* from a positive electrode produces a *positive* deflection on the EKG. A perpendicular wave produces a *biphasic wave;* however, the negative deflection of the biphasic wave now *precedes* the positive deflection.

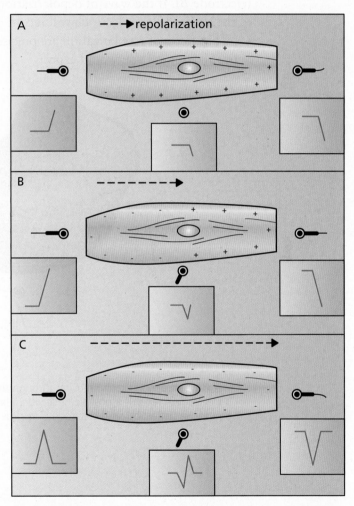

A wave of repolarization moving through muscle tissue is recorded by three different positive electrodes: (*A*) Early repolarization. (*B*) Late repolarization. (*C*) Repolarization is complete.

We can easily apply these concepts to the entire heart. Electrodes placed on the surface of the body will record waves of depolarization and repolarization as they sweep through the heart.

If a wave of depolarization passing through the heart is moving toward a surface electrode, that electrode will record a positive deflection (electrode *A*). If the wave of depolarization is moving away from the electrode, the electrode will record a negative deflection (electrode *B*). If the wave of depolarization is moving perpendicularly to the electrode, the electrode will record a biphasic wave (electrode *C*). The effects of repolarization are precisely the opposite of those of depolarization, as you would expect.

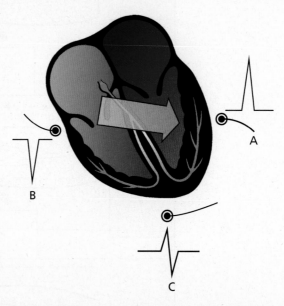

A wave of depolarization moving through the heart (*large arrow*). Electrode *A* records a positive deflection, electrode *B* records a negative deflection, and electrode *C* records a biphasic wave.

The 12 Views of the Heart

If the heart were as simple as a single myocardial cell, a couple of recording electrodes would give us all the information we need to describe its electrical activity. However, as we have already seen, the heart is *not* so simple—a burden to you, a boon to authors of EKG books.

The heart is a three-dimensional organ, and its electrical activity must be understood in three dimensions as well. A couple of electrodes are not adequate to do this, a fact that the original electrocardiographers recognized well over a century ago when they devised the first limb leads. Today, the standard EKG consists of 12 leads, with each lead determined by the placement and orientation of various electrodes on the body. Each lead views the heart at a unique angle, enhancing its sensitivity to a particular region of the heart at the expense of others. The more views, the more information provided.

To read an EKG and extract as much information as possible, you need to understand the 12-lead system.

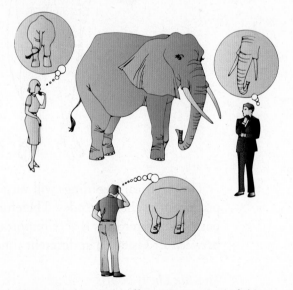

Three observers get three very different impressions of this consummate example of the *Loxodonta africana*. One observer sees the trunk, another sees the body, and the third sees the tail. If you wanted the best description of the elephant, who would you ask? All three, of course.

To prepare a patient for a 12-lead EKG, two electrodes are placed on the arms and two on the legs. These provide the basis for the six *limb leads*, which include the three *standard leads* and the three *augmented leads* (these terms will make more sense in a moment). Six electrodes are also placed across the chest, forming the six *precordial leads*.

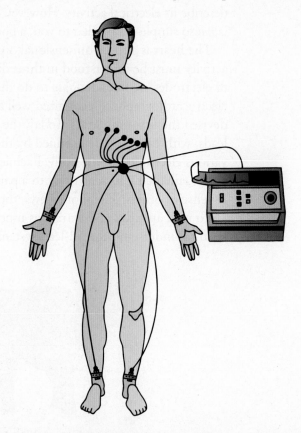

The electrical recordings will vary depending on the precise placement of the electrodes. Therefore, adherence to standard positioning protocols is very important to allow comparison between EKGs taken at different times in different settings.

The Six Limb Leads

The limb leads view the heart in a vertical plane called the *frontal plane*. The frontal plane can be envisioned as a giant circle superimposed on the patient's body. This circle is then marked off in degrees. The limb leads view electrical forces (waves of depolarization and repolarization) moving up and down and left and right through this circle.

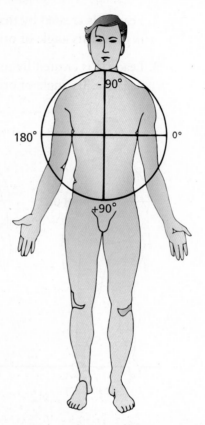

The frontal plane is a coronal plane. The limb leads view electrical forces moving up and down and left and right on the frontal plane.

To produce the six leads of the frontal plane, each of the electrodes is variably designated as positive or negative (this is done automatically by circuitry inside the EKG machine).

Each lead has its own specific view of the heart, or *angle of orientation*. The angle of each lead can be determined by drawing a line from the negative electrode(s) to the positive electrode(s). The resultant angle is then expressed in degrees by superimposing it on the 360° circle of the frontal plane.

The three standard limb leads are defined as follows:

1. Lead I is created by making the left arm positive and the right arm negative. Its angle of orientation is 0°.

2. Lead II is created by making the legs positive and the right arm negative. Its angle of orientation is 60°.

3. Lead III is created by making the legs positive and the left arm negative. Its angle of orientation is 120°.

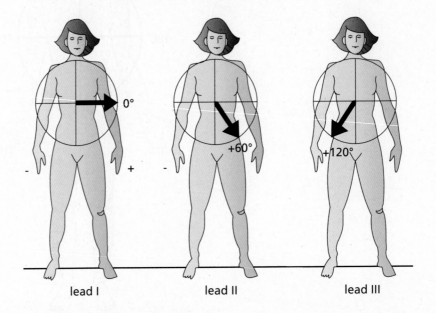

lead I   lead II   lead III

The three augmented limb leads are created somewhat differently. A single lead is chosen to be positive, and all the others are made negative, with their average essentially serving as the negative electrode (common ground). They are called *augmented leads* because the EKG machinery must amplify the tracings to get an adequate recording.

1. Lead aVL is created by making the left arm positive and the other limbs negative. Its angle of orientation is –30°.

2. Lead aVR is created by making the right arm positive and the other limbs negative. Its angle of orientation is –150°.

3. Lead aVF is created by making the legs positive and the other limbs negative. Its angle of orientation is +90°.

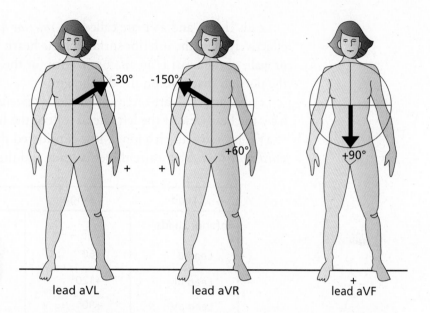

lead aVL   lead aVR   lead aVF

In the next figure, all six leads of the frontal plane are indicated with their appropriate angles of orientation. Just as our three observers each looked at the elephant from his or her own unique perspective, each lead perceives the heart from its own unique point of view.

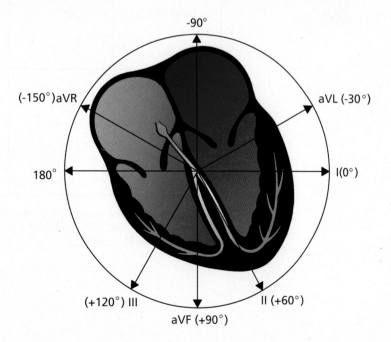

Leads II, III, and aVF are called the *inferior leads* because they most effectively view the inferior surface of the heart. The inferior surface, or wall, of the heart is an anatomic term for the bottom of the heart, the portion that rests on the diaphragm.

Leads I and aVL are often called the *left lateral leads* because they have the best view of the left lateral wall of the heart.

aVR is pretty much a loner. It is considered the only true *right-sided limb lead*. Memorize these six leads and their angles.

Lead	Angle	
Inferior Leads		
Lead II	+60°	
Lead III	+120°	
Lead aVF	+90°	
Left Lateral Leads		
Lead I	+0°	
Lead aVL	-30°	
Right-sided Lead		
Lead aVR	-150°	

Of six limb leads, three are standard (I, II, and III), and three are augmented (aVR, aVL, and aVF). Each lead views the heart from its own particular angle of orientation.

The Six Precordial Leads

The six precordial leads, or chest leads, are even easier to understand. They are arranged across the chest in a *horizontal plane* as illustrated below. Whereas the leads of the frontal plane view electrical forces moving up and down and left and right, the precordial leads record forces moving anteriorly and posteriorly.

To create the six precordial leads, each chest electrode is made positive in turn, and the whole body is taken as the common ground. The six positive electrodes, creating the precordial leads V1 through V6, are positioned as follows:

- V1 is placed in the fourth intercostal space to the right of the sternum.

- V2 is placed in the fourth intercostal space to the left of the sternum.

- V3 is placed between V2 and V4.

- V4 is placed in the fifth intercostal space in the midclavicular line.

- V5 is placed between V4 and V6.

- V6 is placed in the fifth intercostal space in the midaxillary line.

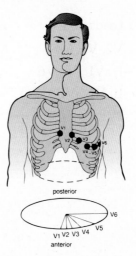

The precordial leads define a horizontal or transverse plane and view electrical forces moving anteriorly and posteriorly.

Just like the limb leads, each precordial lead has its own particular line of sight and region of the heart that it views best.

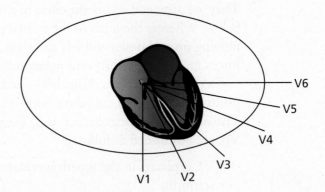

Note that the right ventricle lies anteriorly and medially within the body cavity, and the left ventricle lies posteriorly and laterally. Lead V1 lies directly over the right ventricle, V2 and V3 over the interventricular septum, V4 over the apex of the left ventricle, and V5 and V6 over the lateral left ventricle.

Leads V2 through V4 are often referred to as the *anterior leads,* V5 and V6 join I and aVL as *left lateral leads,* and leads aVR and V1 are the *right ventricular leads.*

Leads	Group
V2, V3, V4	Anterior
I, aVL, V5,V6	Left lateral
II, III, aVF	Inferior
aVR, V1	Right ventricular

A Word About Vectors

It is important to recognize that each EKG electrode records only the *average* current flow at any given moment. Thus, although tiny swirls of current may simultaneously be going off in every direction, each lead records only the instantaneous average of these forces. In this way, out of chaos, some very simple patterns emerge.

This concept is really quite simple; an analogy may be helpful. During the course of a soccer match, a goalie may kick the ball many different times to various members of his team (or, if our hypothetical goalie is not very good, the other team). Some balls will go left, others right, still others straight down the field. However, by the end of the game, the *average direction* of all of the goalie's kicks and tosses is likely to be straight ahead, toward the opposing net. This average movement can be represented by a single arrow, or *vector*.

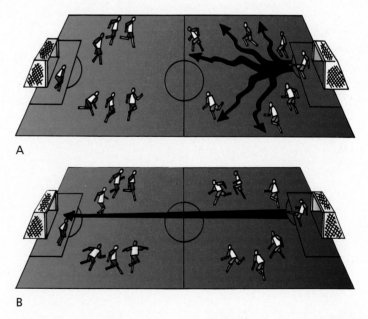

(*A*) The directions of each of the goalie's kicks during the course of the game. (*B*) A single vector represents the average direction and distance of all of these kicks.

This vector is precisely what our EKG electrodes record when measuring the electrical flow within the heart. The vector's angle of orientation represents the average *direction* of current flow, and its length represents the voltage (*amplitude*) attained.

At any given moment, the electrical forces moving within the heart can be represented by a single vector (corresponding to a single kick by the goalie). Furthermore, over any particular period of time during the cardiac cycle (*e.g.*, atrial depolarization), these individual vectors can be summed into a kind of *vector of vectors,* which describes the average direction and magnitude of current flow during that time (*i.e.*, during atrial depolarization, corresponding, let us say, to all the goalie's kicks over the first half of the game). Thus, a particular wave (in this case, the wave of atrial depolarization) can be described by a single vector of given direction and magnitude. You will see how this works and how it simplifies our understanding of the 12-lead EKG in the following section.

The Normal 12-Lead EKG

You now know the three things necessary to derive the normal 12-lead EKG:

1. The normal pathway of cardiac electrical activation and the names of the segments, waves, and intervals that are generated

2. The orientation of all 12 leads, six in the frontal plane and six in the horizontal plane

3. The simple concept that each lead records the average current flow at any given moment

All we need to do now is to take what you already know and figure out what each wave looks like in each of the 12 leads.

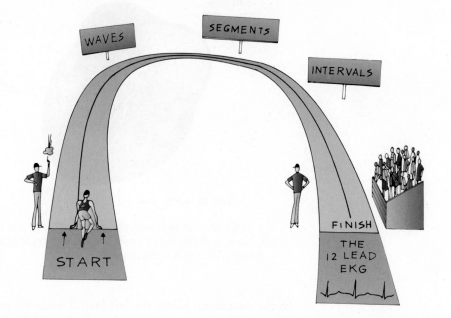

The P Wave

Atrial depolarization begins at the sinus node, high up in the right atrium. The right atrium depolarizes first, then the left atrium. The vector of current flow for atrial depolarization, therefore, points from right to left and slightly inferiorly (*large arrow*).

Any lead that views the wave of atrial depolarization as moving toward it will record a positive deflection on the EKG paper. The left lateral and inferior leads clearly fit this description. In the *frontal plane*, these leads include the left lateral leads I and aVL and the inferior leads II and aVF.

Lead III, which is also one of the inferior leads, is positioned a bit differently. It is the most rightward (orientation +120°) of the inferior leads and actually lies nearly perpendicular to the atrial current. Predictably, lead III frequently records a biphasic P wave.

Lead aVR, the most rightward of all the leads of the frontal plane (orientation −150°), sees the electrical current as moving away; hence, it records a purely negative deflection.

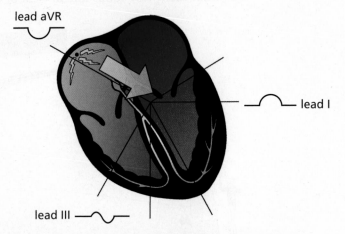

The vector of atrial depolarization points leftward and inferiorly. Therefore, lead I records a positive wave, aVR records a negative wave, and lead III records a biphasic wave.

In the *horizontal plane*, the left lateral leads V5 and V6 record a positive deflection, just as leads I and aVL did in the frontal plane. Lead V1, lying over the right heart, is oriented perpendicularly to the direction of current flow and records a biphasic wave, just like lead III. Leads V2 through V4 are variable.

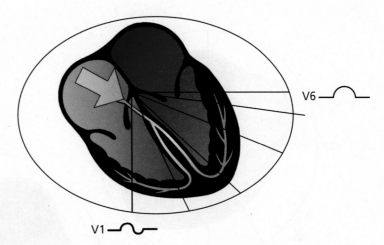

Atrial depolarization in the horizontal plane. V1 records a biphasic wave, and V6 records a positive wave.

Because the atria are small, the voltage they can generate is also small. The amplitude of the P wave does not normally exceed 0.25 mV (2.5 mm, or two and one-half small squares) in any lead. The P wave amplitude is usually most positive in lead II and most negative in lead aVR.

But People Are Individuals

A word of caution is needed. Variations in anatomy and orientation of the heart from person to person make absolute rules impossible. For example, although the P wave in lead III is usually biphasic, it is not uncommon for it to be negative in perfectly normal hearts. All it takes is a change of a few degrees in the vector of current flow to turn a biphasic wave into a negative one. This can happen, for instance, if the patient's heart is angled slightly differently in the chest cavity. For this reason, the normal angle of orientation of current vectors is given in ranges, not precise numbers. For example, the normal range of the P wave vector is 0° to 70°.

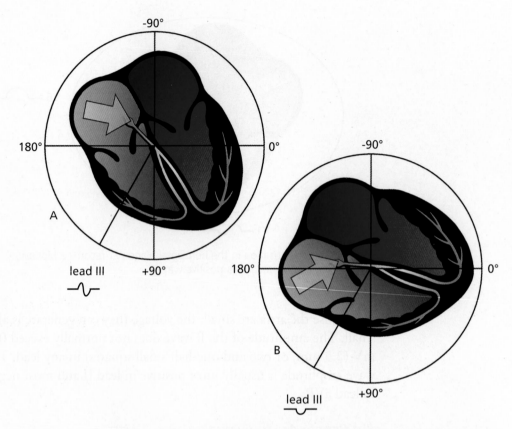

Rotation of the heart within the chest cavity redirects the perceived direction of current flow. Lead III is normally oriented perpendicularly to atrial depolarization. With the apex of the heart turned leftward, lead III will view atrial depolarization as receding and will record a wave that is largely negative.

The PR Interval

The PR interval represents the time from the start of atrial depolarization to the start of ventricular depolarization. It includes the delay in conduction that occurs at the AV node. The PR interval normally lasts from 0.12 to 0.2 seconds (3 to 5 mm on the EKG paper).

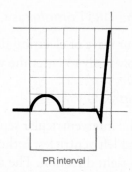

PR interval

The normal PR interval lasts 0.12 to 0.2 seconds.

The PR Segment

The PR segment represents the time from the end of atrial depolarization to the beginning of ventricular depolarization. The PR segment is usually horizontal and runs along the same baseline as the start of the P wave.

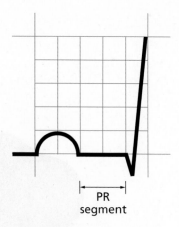

PR segment

The PR segment is horizontal.

The QRS Complex Is Complex, But Not Complicated

Our wave of electrical depolarization, emerging from the AV node, is now ready to enter the ventricles.

Septal Q Waves

The interventricular septum, the wall of muscle separating the right and left ventricles, is the first to depolarize, and it does so in a left-to-right direction. The tiny septal fascicle of the left bundle branch is responsible for rapidly delivering the wave of depolarization to this region of the heart.

Septal depolarization is not always visible on the EKG, but when it is, this small left-to-right depolarization inscribes a tiny negative deflection in one or several of the left lateral leads. This initial negative deflection, or Q wave, may therefore be seen in leads I, aVL, V5, and V6. Sometimes, small Q waves may also be seen in the inferior leads and in V3 and V4.

Normal septal Q waves have an amplitude of not greater than 0.1 mV.

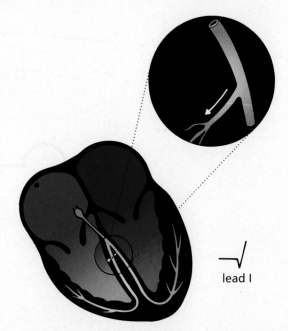

lead I

The left lateral leads view left-to-right septal depolarization as moving away; therefore, they record a small initial negative deflection, or Q wave. Small Q waves are also sometimes seen in the inferior leads; these are normal.

The Rest of the Ventricular Myocardium Depolarizes

The remainder of the ventricles, the vast bulk of the myocardium, depolarizes next. Because the left ventricle is so much more massive than the right ventricle, it dominates the remainder of the QRS complex, and the average vector of current flow swings leftward. Normally, this vector points anywhere from 0° to +90°. In the frontal plane, therefore, large positive deflections (R waves) may be seen in many of the left lateral and inferior leads. Lead aVR, lying rightward, records a deep negative deflection (S wave).

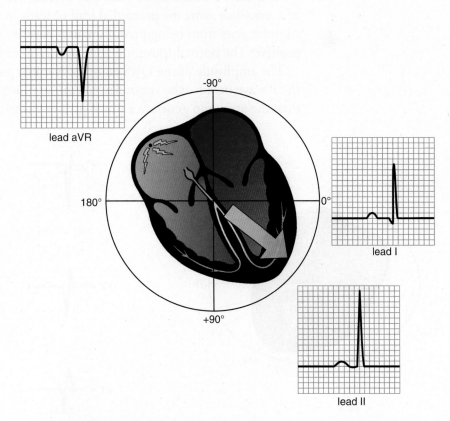

Ventricular depolarization as seen in leads I, II, and aVR. Lead I records a small Q wave due to septal depolarization and a tall R wave. Lead II also records a tall R wave and, less often, a small Q wave. The QRS complex in lead aVR is also deeply negative.

In the horizontal plane, lead V1, which overlies the right ventricle, usually records a deep S wave because the current is moving leftward, away from it. Conversely, leads V5 and V6, lying over the left ventricle, record tall positive R waves. Leads V3 and V4 represent a *transition zone,* and usually, one of these leads records a biphasic wave, that is, an R wave and an S wave of nearly equal amplitude.

This pattern of progressively increasing R wave amplitude moving right to left in the precordial leads is called *R wave progression.* Lead V1 has the smallest R wave; lead V5, the largest (the R wave in lead V6 is usually a little smaller than that in lead V5). We also speak of a *transition zone,* the precordial lead or leads in which the QRS complex goes from being predominantly negative to predominantly positive. The normal transition zone occurs at leads V3 and V4.

The amplitude of the QRS complex is much greater than that of the P wave because the ventricles, having so much more muscle mass than the atria, can generate a much greater electrical potential.

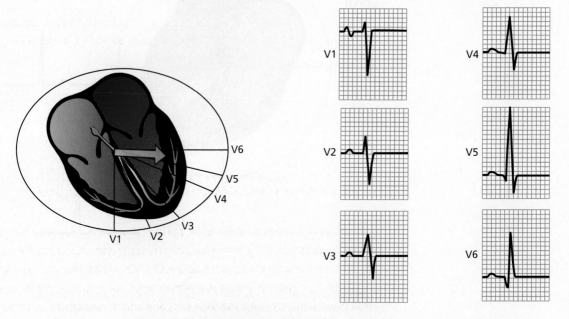

Ventricular depolarization in the precordial leads. Note the normal pattern of R wave progression. The wave in lead V3 is biphasic.

The QRS Interval

A normal QRS interval, representing the duration of the QRS complex, is 0.06 to 0.1 seconds in duration.

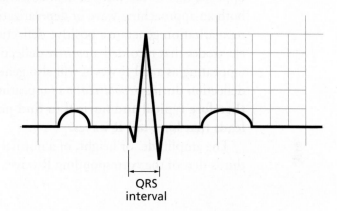

QRS
interval

The ST Segment

The ST segment is usually horizontal or gently upsloping in all leads. It represents the time from the end of ventricular depolarization to the start of ventricular repolarization.

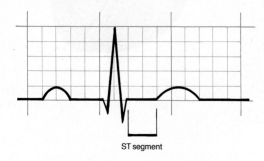

ST segment

The T Wave

The T wave represents ventricular *repolarization*.

   Unlike depolarization, which is largely passive, repolarization requires the expenditure of a great deal of cellular energy (remember the membrane pump). The T wave is highly susceptible to all kinds of influences, both cardiac and noncardiac (*e.g.*, hormonal, neurologic), and is therefore variable in its appearance.

Nevertheless, certain general statements can be made. In the normal heart, repolarization usually begins in the last area of the heart to have been depolarized, and then travels backward, in a direction opposite that of the wave of depolarization (*large arrow*). Because both an approaching wave of depolarization and a receding wave of repolarization generate a positive deflection on the EKG, the same electrodes that recorded a *positive* deflection during *depolarization* (appearing as a tall R wave) will also generally record a *positive* deflection during *repolarization* (appearing as a positive T wave). **It is therefore typical and normal to find positive T waves in the same leads that have tall R waves.**

The amplitude, or height, of a normal T wave is one-third to two-thirds that of the corresponding R wave.

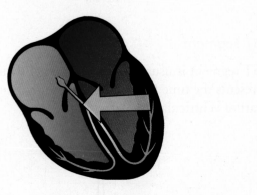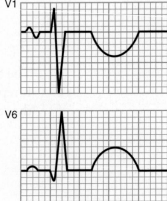

Ventricular repolarization generates a T wave on the EKG. The T wave is usually positive in leads with tall R waves.

The QT Interval

The QT interval encompasses the time from the beginning of ventricular depolarization to the end of ventricular repolarization. It therefore includes all of the electrical events that take place in the ventricles. From the standpoint of time, more of the QT interval is devoted to ventricular *repolarization* than depolarization (*i.e.,* the T wave is wider than the QRS complex).

The duration of the QT interval is proportionate to the heart rate. The faster the heart beats, the faster it must repolarize to prepare for the next contraction; thus, the shorter the QT interval. Conversely, when the heart is beating slowly, there is little urgency to repolarize, and the QT interval is long. In general, the QT interval comprises about 40% of the normal cardiac cycle, as measured from one R wave to the next.

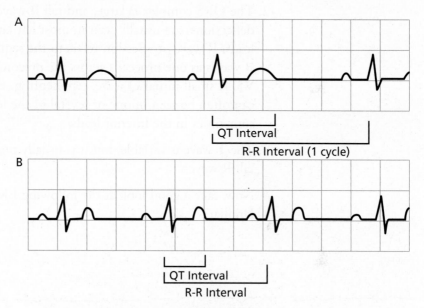

The QT interval composes about 40% of each cardiac cycle (R-R interval). The faster the heart beats, the shorter the QT interval. The heart rate in B is considerably faster than that in A, and the QT interval is correspondingly much shorter (less than one and one-half boxes versus two full boxes).

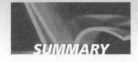

Orientation of the Waves of the Normal EKG

1. The P wave is small and usually positive in the left lateral and inferior leads. It is often biphasic in leads III and V1. It is usually most positive in lead II and most negative in lead aVR.

2. The QRS complex is large, and tall R waves (positive deflections) are usually seen in most left lateral and inferior leads. R wave progression refers to the sequential enlargement of R waves as one proceeds across the precordial leads from V1 to V5. A small initial Q wave, representing septal depolarization, can often be seen in one or several of the left lateral leads, and sometimes in the inferior leads.

3. The T wave is variable, but it is usually positive in leads with tall R waves.

4. Now, take a good look at the following EKG. Does it seem familiar?

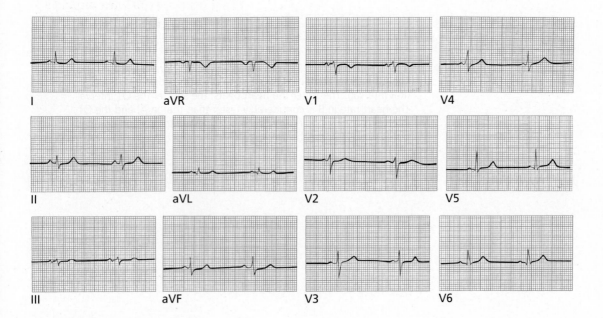

Of course it seems familiar. It's a normal 12-lead EKG, identical to the one that began the book.

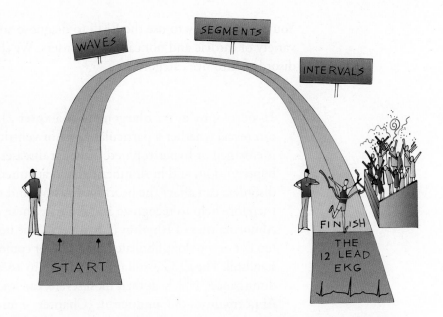

Congratulations! You have successfully traversed the most difficult terrain in this book. Everything that follows builds logically from the few basic principles you have just mastered.

Coming Attractions

You are now ready to use the EKG to diagnose an extraordinary variety of cardiac and noncardiac disorders. We shall group these disorders into five categories.

Hypertrophy and Enlargement (Chapter 2). The EKG can reveal whether a particular atrial or ventricular chamber is enlarged or hypertrophied. Valvular diseases, sustained hypertension, and both inherited and acquired cardiac muscle disorders can affect the heart in this way, and the EKG can therefore help to recognize and evaluate these disorders.

Abnormalities of Rhythm (Chapter 3). The heart can beat too fast or too slow, fibrillate chaotically, or come to a sudden standstill. The EKG is still the best means to assess such rhythm disturbances, which, at their most severe, can lead to sudden death.

Abnormalities of Conduction (Chapters 4 and 5). If the normal pathways of cardiac electrical conduction become blocked, the heart rate can fall precipitously. The result can be syncope, a faint caused by a sudden decrease in cardiac output. Syncope is one of the leading causes of hospital admission. Conduction can also be accelerated along short circuits that bypass the normal delay in the AV node; we will look at these, too.

Myocardial Ischemia and Infarction (Chapter 6). The diagnosis of myocardial ischemia and infarction is one of the most important roles for the EKG. There are many reasons why a patient may have chest pain, and the EKG can help sort these out.

Electrolyte Disturbances, Drug Effects, and Miscellaneous Disorders (Chapter 7). Because all of the electrical events of the heart are dependent on electrolytes, it stands to reason that various electrolyte disorders can affect cardiac conduction and even lead to sudden death if untreated. Medications such as digitalis, antidepressants, antiarrhythmic agents, and even antibiotics can profoundly alter the EKG. A number of cardiac and noncardiac diseases can also cause dramatic shifts in the EKG. In each of these instances, a timely glance at an EKG may be diagnostic and sometimes lifesaving.

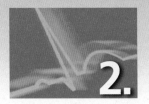

2. Hypertrophy and Enlargement of the Heart

In this chapter you will learn:

1 what happens to a wave on the EKG when an atrium enlarges or a ventricle hypertrophies

2 the meaning of electrical axis and its importance in diagnosing hypertrophy and enlargement

3 the criteria for the EKG diagnosis of right and left atrial enlargement

4 the criteria for the EKG diagnosis of right and left ventricular hypertrophy

5 about the cases of Mildred W. and Tom L., which will test your ability to recognize the EKG changes of hypertrophy and enlargement.

Definitions

The term *hypertrophy* refers to an increase in muscle mass. The wall of a hypertrophied ventricle is thick and powerful. Most hypertrophy is caused by *pressure overload,* in which the heart is forced to pump blood against an increased resistance, as in patients with systemic hypertension or aortic stenosis. Just as weight lifters develop powerful pectoral muscles as they bench press progressively heavier and heavier weights, so the heart muscle grows thicker and stronger as it is called on to eject blood against increasing resistance.

Enlargement refers to dilatation of a particular chamber. An enlarged ventricle can hold more blood than a normal ventricle. Enlargement is typically caused by *volume overload:* the chamber dilates to accommodate an increased amount of blood. Enlargement is most often seen with certain valvular diseases. Aortic insufficiency, for example, may cause left ventricular enlargement, and mitral insufficiency may result in left atrial enlargement.

Enlargement and hypertrophy frequently coexist. This is not surprising because both represent ways in which the heart tries to increase its cardiac output.

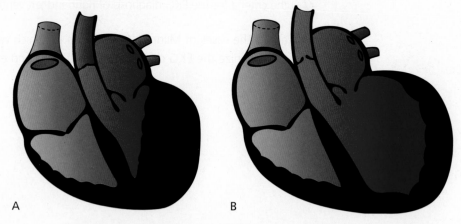

A   B

(*A*) A hypertrophied left ventricle caused by aortic stenosis. The wall is so thick that the chamber size is actually diminished. (*B*) An enlarged left ventricle. The chamber is bigger, but the wall thickness is normal.

The EKG is not very good at distinguishing between hypertrophy and enlargement. However, it is traditional to speak of *atrial enlargement* and *ventricular hypertrophy* when reading EKGs.*

Because the P wave represents atrial depolarization, we look at the P wave to assess atrial enlargement. Similarly, we examine the QRS complex to determine whether there is ventricular hypertrophy.

*The term atrial enlargement has been supplanted in the minds of some by the term atrial abnormalities. This change in terminology reflects the recognition that a variety of electrical abnormalities can cause the changes on the EKG characteristically associated with atrial enlargement. However, we will continue to use the term atrial enlargement in this book, both because the term is more rooted in tradition (and traditional values still matter as we race headlong through the new millennium) and because the vast majority of cases of P wave changes are due to enlargement of the atria.

How the EKG Can Change

Three things can happen to a wave on the EKG when a chamber hypertrophies or enlarges:

1. The chamber can take longer to depolarize. The EKG wave may therefore *increase in duration.*

2. The chamber can generate more current and thus a larger voltage. The wave may therefore *increase in amplitude.*

3. A larger percentage of the total electrical current can move through the expanded chamber. The mean electrical vector, or what we call the *electrical axis,* of the EKG wave may therefore shift.

Because the concept of axis is so important for diagnosing hypertrophy and enlargement, we need to digress for just a moment to elaborate on this idea.

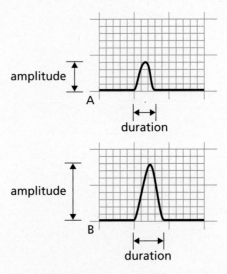

(*A*) A normal wave. (*B*) The same wave when the chamber has enlarged or hypertrophied. The amplitude and duration of the wave have increased. A third alteration, a shift in the electrical axis, is discussed in the following pages.

Axis

Earlier, we discussed how the EKG records the instantaneous vector of electrical forces at any given moment. Using this idea, we can represent the complete depolarization (or repolarization) of a chamber by drawing a series of sequential vectors, each vector representing the sum of all the electrical forces at a given moment.

Because it is easier to visualize, let's first look at ventricular depolarization (the QRS complex) before turning to atrial depolarization (the P wave) and ventricular repolarization (the T wave).

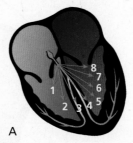

A

Ventricular depolarization is represented by eight sequential instantaneous vectors, illustrating how the electrical forces normally move progressively leftward. Although, for the sake of clarity, we have shown only eight instantaneous vectors, we could just as well have shown 18 or 8,000.

The first vector represents septal depolarization, and each successive vector represents progressive depolarization of the ventricles. The vectors swing progressively leftward because the electrical activity of the much larger left ventricle increasingly dominates the EKG.

The average vector of all of the instantaneous vectors is called the *mean vector*.

The *direction* of the mean vector is called the **mean electrical axis.**

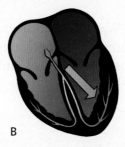

B

A single vector summarizes all of the instantaneous vectors. This summation vector is called the mean vector, and its direction is the axis of ventricular depolarization. Axis is defined in the frontal plane only.

The mean QRS vector points leftward and inferiorly, representing the average direction of current flow during ventricular depolarization. The normal QRS axis—the direction of this mean vector—thus lies between +90° and 0°. (Actually, most cardiologists extend the range of normal from +90° to –30°. In time, as you become more comfortable with the concept of axis, you should add this refinement to your electrical analysis, but for now +90° to 0° is satisfactory.)

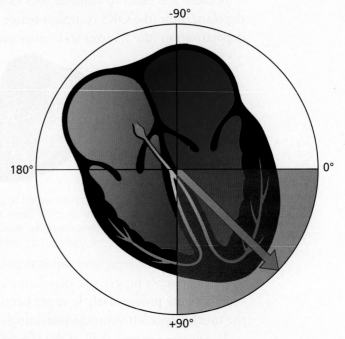

If the QRS axis lies within the shaded quadrant, between 0° and 90°, it is normal.

We can quickly determine whether the QRS axis on any EKG is normal by looking only at leads I and aVF. **If the QRS complex is positive in leads I and aVF, the QRS axis must be normal.** Why is this?

Determining Whether the QRS Axis Is Normal

We know that any lead will record a positive deflection if the wave of depolarization is moving toward it. Lead I is oriented at 0°. Thus, if the mean QRS vector is directed anywhere between –90° and +90°, lead I will record a predominantly positive QRS complex.

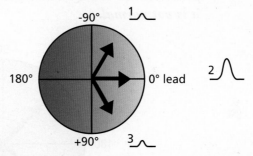

Any mean QRS vector oriented between –90° and +90° will produce a predominantly positive QRS complex in lead I. Three different QRS mean vectors are shown. All three are oriented between –90° and +90°; hence, they will all produce a predominantly positive QRS complex. The three QRS complexes depicted here illustrate what lead I would record for each of the three vectors.

Lead aVF is oriented at +90°. If the mean QRS vector is directed anywhere between 0° and 180°, lead aVF will record a predominantly positive QRS complex.

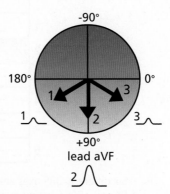

Any mean QRS vector oriented between 0° and 180° will produce a predominantly positive QRS complex in lead aVF. Three different mean QRS vectors are shown, all oriented so that lead aVF will record a predominantly positive deflection as illustrated.

If the QRS complex is predominantly positive in *both* lead I and lead aVF, then the QRS axis must lie in the quadrant where both are positive, that is, between 0° and +90°. This is the normal QRS axis.

Another way to look at this is to take the converse approach: **if the QRS complex in either lead I or lead aVF is *not predominantly positive,* then the QRS axis does not lie between 0° and +90°, and it is *not normal.***

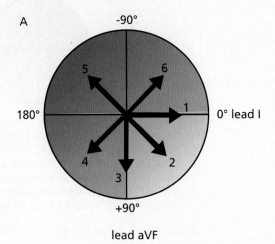

Six different QRS axes are shown (*A*). Only an axis directed between 0° and +90° (*shaded quadrant*) will produce a predominantly positive QRS complex in both lead I and lead aVF. (*B*) The QRS complexes in leads I and aVF associated with each of the six axes are shown. Only axis 2 is normal and associated with a predominantly positive QRS complex in both leads, although most cardiologists would consider axis 1 and axis 3 to be normal as well.

Defining the Axis Precisely

Although it is usually sufficient to note whether the axis is normal or not, it is possible to be more rigorous and to define the actual angle of the axis with fair precision. All you need to do is look for the limb lead in which the QRS complex is most nearly **biphasic**, that is, with equal positive and negative deflections (sometimes the deflections are so small that the wave appears flat, or **isoelectric**). The axis must then be oriented approximately **perpendicular** to this lead because an electrode oriented perpendicularly to the mean direction of current flow records a biphasic wave.

Thus, for example, if the QRS complex in lead III (orientation, +120°) is biphasic, then the axis must be oriented at right angles (90°) to this lead, at either +30° or –150°. And, if we already know that the axis is normal—that is, if the QRS complex is positive in leads I and aVF—then the axis cannot be –150°, but must be +30°.

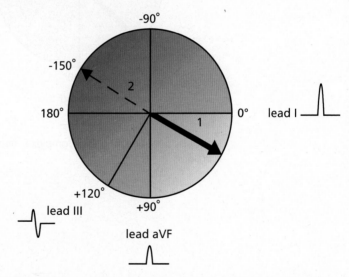

QRS complexes are shown for leads I, III, and aVF. Determining the axis is easy. The QRS complex in lead III is biphasic. The axis therefore must be either +30° or −150°. However, because the QRS complex is positive in both leads I and aVF, the axis must be normal; that is, it must lie within the shaded quadrant. The axis therefore can only be +30°.

Axis Deviation: Getting More Specific About Defining Abnormal Axes

The normal QRS axis is between 0° and 90°. If the axis lies between 90° and 180°, we speak of *right axis deviation*. Will the QRS complex in leads I and aVF be positive or negative in a patient with right axis deviation?

The QRS complex in lead aVF will still be positive, but it will be negative in lead I.

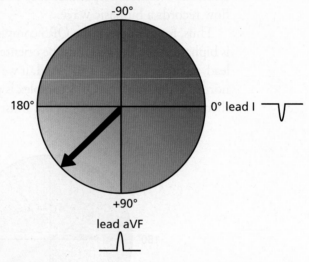

Right axis deviation. The QRS complex is negative in lead I, whereas it is positive in aVF.

If the axis lies between 0° and –90°, we speak *of left axis deviation*. In this case, the QRS complex in lead I will be positive, but it will be negative in lead aVF.

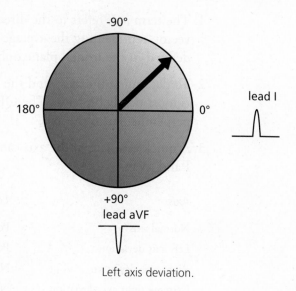

Left axis deviation.

In rare instances, the axis becomes totally disoriented and lies between –90° and 180°. This is called *extreme right axis deviation*. The QRS complex in both lead aVF and lead I will be negative.

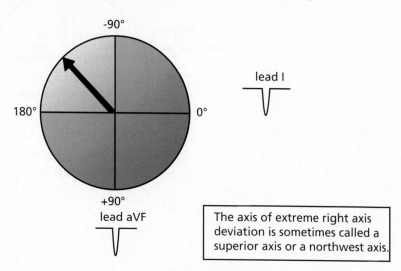

The axis of extreme right axis deviation is sometimes called a superior axis or a northwest axis.

Extreme right axis deviation.

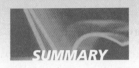

SUMMARY   Axis

1. The term *axis* refers to the direction of the mean electrical vector, representing the average direction of current flow. It is defined in the frontal plane only.

2. To determine the axis, find the lead in which the QRS complex is most nearly biphasic. The QRS axis must lie approximately perpendicular to the axis.

3. A quick estimate of the axis can be made by looking at leads I and aVF:

Axis	Lead I	Lead aVF
Normal axis	Positive	Positive
Left axis deviation	Positive	Negative
Right axis deviation	Negative	Positive
Extreme right axis deviation	Negative	Negative

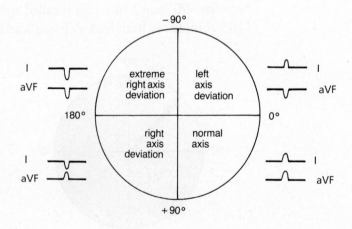

On the EKG below, the waves recorded by the six leads of the frontal plane are shown. Is the QRS axis normal, or is there axis deviation?

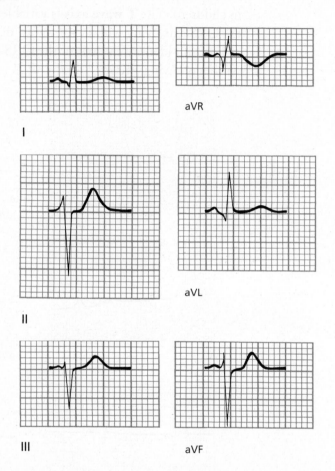

This patient has left axis deviation; the QRS complex is predominantly positive in lead I and negative in lead aVF.

Now, can you define the axis more precisely by finding the lead with a biphasic QRS complex?

The QRS complex in lead aVR is approximately biphasic; therefore, the electrical axis must lie nearly perpendicular to it, that is, at either –60° or +120°. Because we already know that the axis falls within the zone of left axis deviation (*i.e.,* between 0° and –90°), the correct axis must be –60°.

Just as we have done for the QRS complex, so we can define an axis for the P wave and T wave on every EKG. The normal **P wave axis** lies approximately between 0° and 70° in adults (between 0° and 90° in children). The **T wave axis** is variable, but it should approximate the QRS axis, lying within 50° to 60° of the QRS axis.

Can you identify the axis of the QRS complex, P wave, and T wave on the following EKG?

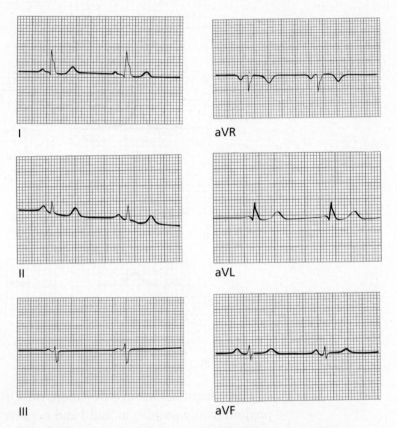

(A) The QRS axis is about 0°. It is nearly biphasic in aVF, implying an axis of 0° or 180°. Because the QRS complex in lead I has a tall R wave, the axis must be 0°. (B) Lead aVL is nearly isoelectric for the P wave, so the P wave axis must be either 60° or −120°. Since the P wave is positive in leads I and aVF, the axis must be 60°. (C) All of the leads with tall R waves have positive T waves. The T waves are flat in lead III, indicating an axis perpendicular to lead III (either + 30° or −150°). Because there is a tall T wave in lead I, the axis must be about +30°.

Axis Deviation, Hypertrophy, and Enlargement

Why does axis deviation have anything to do with hypertrophy and enlargement? Because the concept of axis deviation is most successfully applied to ventricular hypertrophy, let's consider what happens to the flow of electricity when a ventricle hypertrophies.

In the normal heart, the QRS axis lies between 0° and +90°, reflecting the electrical dominance of the much larger left ventricle over the right ventricle. Imagine, now, a 65-year-old man who has allowed his hypertension to go untreated for many years. He comes to see you for headaches and shortness of breath, and you discover a greatly elevated blood pressure of 190/115 mm Hg. This sustained and severe hypertension has forced the left ventricle to work too hard for too long, and it has hypertrophied. Its electrical dominance over the right ventricle has therefore become even more profound. The mean electrical vector is drawn even further leftward, and the result is *left axis deviation*.

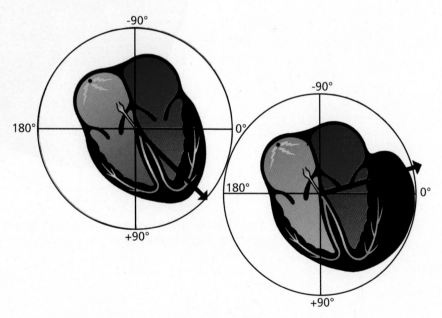

With left ventricular hypertrophy, the electrical axis moves further leftward, resulting in left axis deviation.

Right ventricular hypertrophy is far less common and requires a huge change in the proportions of the right ventricle in order to overcome the electrical forces generated by the normally dominant left ventricle. It can occur, however, in patients with chronic obstructive pulmonary disease sufficiently severe to cause pulmonary artery hypertension or in patients with uncorrected congenital heart disease associated with profound volume or pressure overload of the right ventricle. If the right ventricle greatly hypertrophies, it can be detected on the EKG as a shift in the QRS axis. The mean electrical axis of current flow is drawn rightward, and the result is *right axis deviation.*

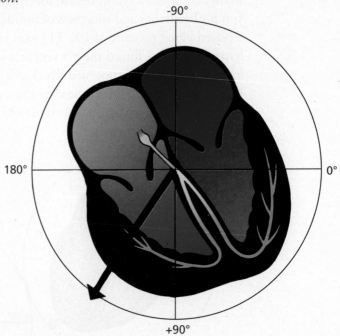

With right ventricular hypertrophy, the electrical axis moves rightward, resulting in right axis deviation.

This is a good time to restate the three things that can happen to a wave on the EKG with enlargement or hypertrophy:

1. The wave can increase in duration.
2. The wave can increase in amplitude.
3. The electrical axis of the wave can deviate from normal.

Specific EKG criteria for the diagnosis of atrial enlargement and ventricular hypertrophy have been devised, and these are discussed in the following pages.

Atrial Enlargement

The normal P wave is less than 0.12 second in duration, and the largest deflection, whether positive or negative, should not exceed 2.5 mm. The first part of the P wave represents right atrial depolarization and the second part left atrial depolarization.

Virtually all of the information you need to assess atrial enlargement can be found in leads II and V1. Lead II is useful because it is oriented nearly parallel to the flow of current through the atria (*i.e.*, parallel to the mean P wave vector). It therefore records the largest positive deflection and is very sensitive to any perturbations in atrial depolarization. Lead V1 is useful because it is oriented perpendicularly to the flow of electricity and is therefore biphasic, allowing easy separation of the right and left atrial components.

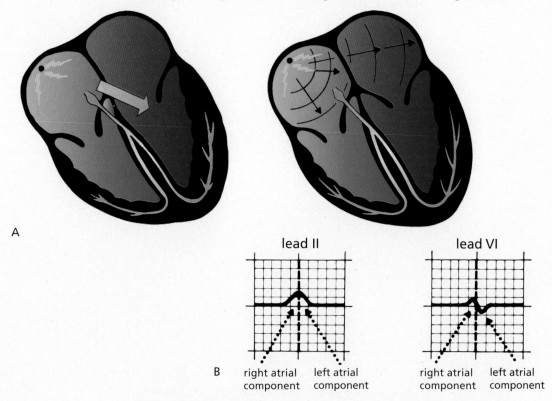

(*A*) Normal atrial depolarization. (*B*) The normal P wave in leads II and V1. The first part of the P wave represents right atrial depolarization, and the second part represents left atrial depolarization.

Right Atrial Enlargement

With *right atrial enlargement,* the amplitude of the first portion of the P wave increases. The width does not change because the terminal component of the P wave is *left* atrial in origin, and this remains unchanged.

Enlargement of the right atrium may also cause the right atrium to dominate the left atrium electrically. The vector of atrial depolarization may swing rightward, and the P wave axis may move rightward toward or even beyond +90°. The tallest P wave may therefore no longer appear in lead II, but in lead aVF or lead III.

The classic picture of right atrial enlargement is illustrated in leads II and V1, below, and has been called *P pulmonale* because it is often caused by severe lung disease.

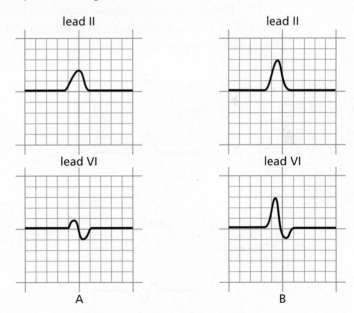

(*A*) The normal P wave in leads II and V1. (*B*) Right atrial enlargement. Note the increased amplitude of the early, right atrial component of the P wave. The terminal left atrial component, and hence the overall duration of the P wave, are essentially unchanged.

Right atrial enlargement is diagnosed by the presence of P waves with an amplitude exceeding 2.5 mm in the inferior leads II, III, and aVF.

Left Atrial Enlargement

With *left atrial enlargement,* the second portion of the P wave may increase in amplitude. The diagnosis of left atrial enlargement requires that the terminal (left atrial) portion of the P wave should drop more than 1 mm below the isoelectric line in lead V1.

However, a more prominent change in the P wave is an increase in its *duration.* This occurs because left atrial depolarization represents the terminal portion of the P wave, and prolonged depolarization can be readily seen (with *right* atrial enlargement, prolonged depolarization of the right atrium is hidden by the left atrial portion of the P wave). The diagnosis of left atrial enlargement, therefore, also requires that the terminal portion of the P wave should be at least 1 small block (0.04 second) in width.

The electrocardiographic picture of left atrial enlargement has been called *P mitrale* because mitral valve disease is a common cause of left atrial enlargement.

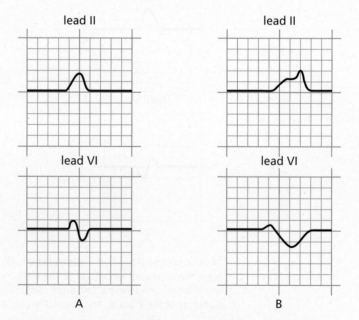

(*A*) Again, the normal P wave in leads II and V1. (*B*) Left atrial enlargement. Note the increased amplitude and duration of the terminal, left atrial component of the P wave.

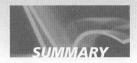
SUMMARY

Atrial Enlargement

To diagnose atrial enlargement, look at leads II and V1.

Right atrial enlargement is characterized by the following:

1. P waves with an amplitude exceeding 2.5 mm in the inferior leads

2. No change in the duration of the P wave

3. Possible right axis deviation of the P wave.

Left atrial enlargement is characterized by the following:

1. The amplitude of the terminal (negative) component of the P wave may be increased and must descend at least 1 mm below the isoelectric line in lead V1.

2. The duration of the P wave is increased, and the terminal (negative) portion of the P wave must be at least 1 small block (0.04 second) in width.

3. No significant axis deviation is seen because the left atrium is normally electrically dominant.

It should be stressed again that electrocardiographic evidence of atrial enlargement (especially left atrial enlargement) often has no pathologic correlate and may in some cases merely reflect some nonspecific conduction abnormality. Abnormalities of the P wave axis can also be seen when the heart rhythm arises from a source other than the sinus node, something we shall discuss later. Interpretation of atrial enlargement on the EKG must therefore be tempered by knowledge of the clinical setting (a good idea in any circumstance!).

Ventricular Hypertrophy

The diagnosis of ventricular hypertrophy requires a careful assessment of the QRS complex in many leads.

Right Ventricular Hypertrophy

Looking at the Limb Leads

In the limb leads, the most common feature associated with right ventricular hypertrophy is right axis deviation; that is, the electrical axis of the QRS complex, normally between 0° and +90°, veers off between +90° and +180°. This reflects the new electrical dominance of the usually electrically submissive right ventricle.

Many cardiologists feel that the QRS axis must exceed +100° in order to make the diagnosis of right ventricular hypertrophy. Therefore, the QRS complex in lead I (oriented at 0°) must be more negative than positive.

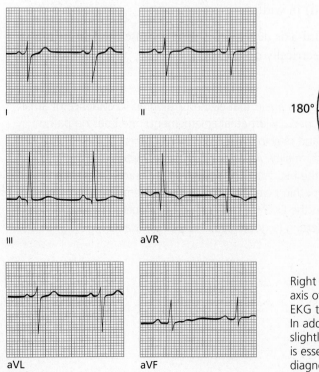

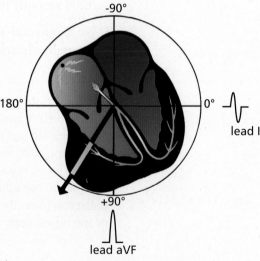

Right ventricular hypertrophy shifts the axis of the QRS complex to the right. The EKG tracings confirm right axis deviation. In addition, the QRS complex in lead I is slightly negative, a criterion that many believe is essential for properly establishing the diagnosis of right ventricular hypertrophy.

Looking at the Precordial Leads

The precordial leads can also be helpful in diagnosing right ventricular hypertrophy. As you might expect, the normal pattern of R wave progression, whereby the R wave amplitude enlarges as you proceed from lead V1 to V5, is disrupted. Instead of the R wave amplitude increasing as the leads move closer to the left ventricle, the reverse may occur. There may be a large R wave in lead V1, which lies over the hypertrophied right ventricle, and a small R wave in leads V5 and V6, which lies over the normal, but now electrically humble, left ventricle. Similarly, the S wave in lead V1 is small, whereas the S wave in lead V6 is large.

These criteria have been expressed in the simplest possible mathematics:

- In lead V1, the R wave is larger than the S wave.

- In lead V6, the S wave is larger than the R wave.

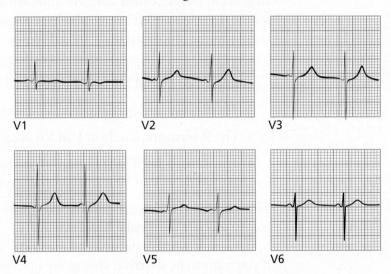

In lead V1, the R wave is larger than the S wave. In lead V6, the S wave is larger than the R wave.

The most common causes of right ventricular hypertrophy are pulmonary disease and congenital heart disease.

Left Ventricular Hypertrophy

The diagnosis of left ventricular hypertrophy is somewhat more complicated. Left axis deviation beyond −15° is often seen, but by and large this is not a very useful diagnostic feature. Instead, **increased R wave amplitude in those leads overlying the left ventricle forms the basis for the EKG diagnosis of left ventricular hypertrophy.**

Unfortunately, there are almost as many criteria for diagnosing left ventricular hypertrophy on the EKG as there are books about EKGs. Nevertheless, all the criteria reflect a common theme: **there should be increased R wave amplitude in leads overlying the left ventricle and increased S wave amplitude in leads overlying the right ventricle.** The various criteria vary in their sensitivity and specificity. Those listed here are not the only ones, but they will serve you well.

Looking at the Precordial Leads

In general, the precordial leads are more sensitive than the limb leads for the diagnosis of left ventricular hypertrophy. The most useful criteria in the precordial leads are as follows:

1. The R wave amplitude in lead V5 or V6 *plus* the S wave amplitude in lead V1 or V2 exceeds 35 mm.

2. The R wave amplitude in lead V5 exceeds 26 mm.

3. The R wave amplitude in lead V6 exceeds 18 mm.

4. The R wave amplitude in lead V6 exceeds the R wave amplitude in lead V5.

The more criteria that are positive, the greater the likelihood that the patient has left ventricular hypertrophy.

It is, sadly, worth your while to memorize all of these criteria, but if you want to be selective, choose the first because it probably has the best predictive value.

> **Note:** These criteria are of little value in individuals younger than 35 years of age, who frequently have increased voltage due, in many cases, to a relatively thin chest wall. They are particularly unreliable in young children.

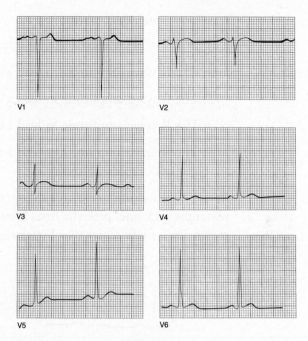

Left ventricular hypertrophy in the precordial leads. Three of the four criteria are met: the R wave amplitude in V5 plus the S wave amplitude in V1 exceeds 35 mm, the R wave amplitude in V6 exceeds 18 mm, and the R wave amplitude in lead V6 slightly exceeds the R wave amplitude in lead V5. The only criterion not met is for the R wave in lead V5 to exceed 26 mm.

Looking at the Limb Leads

The most useful criteria in the limb leads are as follows:

1. The R wave amplitude in lead aVL exceeds 13 mm.

2. The R wave amplitude in lead aVF exceeds 21 mm.

3. The R wave amplitude in lead I exceeds 14 mm.

4. The R wave amplitude in lead I *plus* the S wave amplitude in lead III exceeds 25 mm.

Again, if you aspire to electrocardiographic nirvana, learn them all. If you must pick one, pick the first. However, although it has excellent specificity for left ventricular hypertrophy, it is not very sensitive.

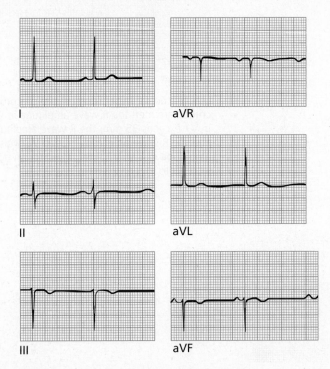

Left ventricular hypertrophy in the limb leads. Criteria 1, 3, and 4 are met; only criterion 2, regarding the R wave amplitude in lead aVF, is not met.

The leading causes of left ventricular hypertrophy are systemic hypertension and valvular disease.

You may have noticed that, in our discussion of ventricular hypertrophy, no comment has been made about the *duration* of the QRS complex. Both right and left ventricular hypertrophy may slightly prolong the QRS complex, but rarely beyond 0.1 second.

When Both Ventricles Are Hypertrophied

What happens when *both* the right ventricle and left ventricle are hypertrophied? As you might expect, there may be a combination of features (*e.g.*, criteria for left ventricular hypertrophy in the precordial leads with right axis deviation in the limb leads), but in most cases, the effects of the usually dominant left ventricle obscure those of the right ventricle.

Is there ventricular hypertrophy in the tracing below?

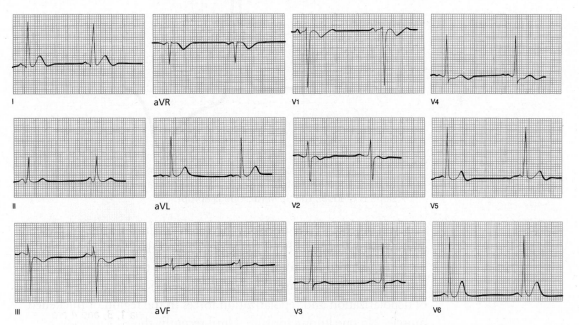

Yes. This patient has aortic stenosis and has left ventricular hypertrophy on the EKG. He meets the criteria in both the precordial and limb leads.

Secondary Repolarization Abnormalities of Ventricular Hypertrophy

Something else may happen with hypertrophy of a ventricle that can dramatically alter the EKG, specifically the ST segment and the T wave. These changes are called *secondary repolarization abnormalities* and include the following:

1. Down-sloping ST segment depression

2. T wave inversion (*i.e.*, the T wave changes its axis so that it is no longer aligned with the QRS axis).

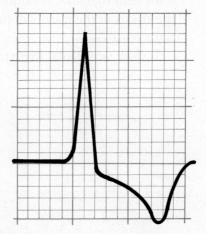

Note how the depressed ST segment and the inverted T wave appear to blend together to form a single asymmetric wave. The downward slope is gradual; the upward slope is abrupt.

Several theories have been advanced to explain the cause of these abnormalities, ranging from inadequate blood flow in the capillary beds of the subendocardium (the inner layer of the myocardium lying just beneath the endocardial lining of the ventricle) to an overlapping of depolarization and repolarization forces in the region of thickened muscle. No one knows for sure. Until recently, these changes were referred to as *strain*, but the implication that these changes necessarily reflect the *straining* of an overworked and hypoxic muscle has proven to be more simplistic than true, and the term should rightly be discarded.

Repolarization abnormalities are not at all uncommon. They are most evident in those leads with tall R waves (reasonably so, because these leads lie over, and most directly reflect, the electrical forces of the hypertrophied ventricle). Thus, right ventricular repolarization abnormalities will be seen in leads V1 and V2, and left ventricular repolarization abnormalities will be most evident in leads I, aVL, V5, and V6. Left ventricular secondary repolarization abnormalities are far more common than right ventricular abnormalities.

Repolarization abnormalities usually accompany severe hypertrophy and may even herald the onset of ventricular dilatation. For example, a patient with aortic stenosis and no clinical symptoms may show a stable pattern of left ventricular hypertrophy for years. Eventually, however, the left ventricle may fail, and the patient will develop severe shortness of breath and other symptoms of congestive heart failure. The EKG may then show left ventricular hypertrophy with secondary repolarization abnormalities. This progression is illustrated in the two EKGs below.

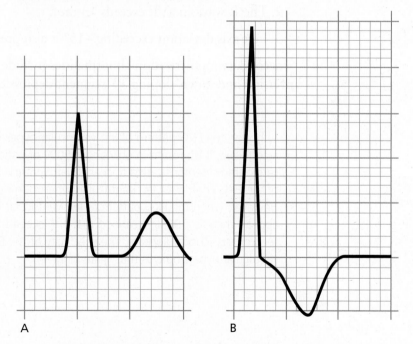

A   B

(*A*) Lead aVL in a patient with aortic stenosis and left ventricular hypertrophy. Note the tall R wave, meeting the criteria for left ventricular hypertrophy. The ST segment is flat, and the T wave is upright. (*B*) One year later, the same lead shows the development of secondary repolarization abnormalities, reflecting the onset of left ventricular failure. The ST segment is depressed, and the T wave is inverted. Note, too, that the amplitude of the R wave has increased.

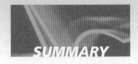

SUMMARY

Ventricular Hypertrophy

Right ventricular hypertrophy is characterized by the following:

1. Right axis deviation is present, with the QRS axis exceeding +100°.

2. The R wave is larger than the S wave in V1, whereas the S wave is larger than the R wave in V6.

Left ventricular hypertrophy is characterized by voltage criteria and, not infrequently, secondary repolarization abnormalities. The two most useful voltage criteria are the following:

1. The R wave in V5 or V6 plus the S wave in V1 or V2 exceeds 35 mm.

2. The R wave in aVL exceeds 13 mm.

3. Left axis deviation exceeding –15° is also present.

Secondary repolarization abnormalities include asymmetric, T wave inversion and down-sloping ST segment depression.

Although the EKG pattern of left ventricular hypertrophy is easily recognized, it is present in only about 50% of patients whose echo-cardiograms demonstrate a thickened left ventricle. The sensitivity of the EKG criteria for left ventricular hypertrophy is thus fairly low. However, when the EKG pattern of left ventricular hypertrophy does appear, there is a 90% likelihood that a thickened ventricle will be seen on an echocardiogram. The specificity of the EKG criteria for left ventricular hypertrophy is thus quite high.

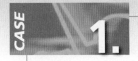

CASE 1.

Mildred W., a 53-year-old widow (her husband died of cerebral anoxia induced by his futile efforts to memorize all of the EKG criteria for left ventricular hypertrophy), comes to your office for a routine checkup. She is new to your practice and has not seen a doctor since her last child was born, which was more than 20 years ago. She has no specific complaints other than an occasional sinus headache. Routine physical examination is unremarkable, except that you find her blood pressure is 170/110 mm Hg. She is unaware of being hypertensive. You would like to know if her hypertension is long-standing or of recent onset. Your laboratory assessment includes measurement of serum electrolytes, creatinine, and blood urea nitrogen; urinalysis; chest x-ray; and the EKG shown below. Is the EKG helpful?

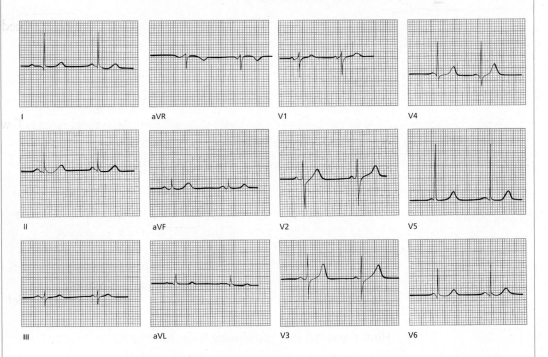

Mildred's EKG is essentially normal, which is not at all surprising. Most patients with hypertension have normal EKGs. Nevertheless, had you found left ventricular hypertrophy, with or without repolarization abnormalities, you would have had at least one piece of evidence suggesting that her hypertension is long-standing. In this particular case, a cardiac echogram could be done to exclude hypertrophy, but it is certainly not necessary in order to decide that Mildred should be treated.

CASE

2.

Tom L. is a 23-year-old marathon runner. Topping Heartbreak Hill at about the 20-mile mark of the New York Marathon, he suddenly turns pale, clutches his chest, and drops to the ground. Another runner, although on pace for a personal best, stops to help. Finding Tom pulseless and apneic, he begins cardiopulmonary resuscitation. The timely intervention proves lifesaving. Tom responds, and moments later the following EKG is taken as he is being rushed to the nearest hospital. Why did Tom collapse?

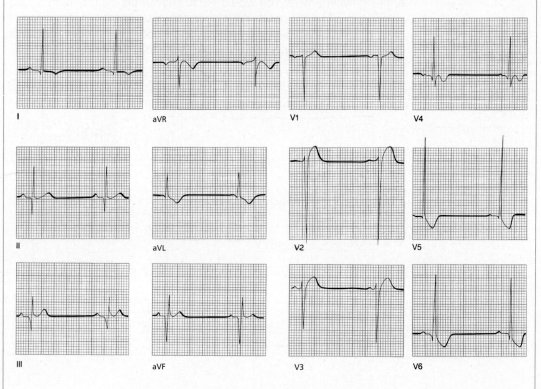

I   aVR   V1   V4

II   aVL   V2   V5

III   aVF   V3   V6

Hint: If you get this, you already know too much.

Tom L. collapsed because of a hypertrophic disease of his heart muscle. A leading cause of sudden death in young, healthy athletes is hypertrophic cardiomyopathy, of which one variant is **hypertrophic obstructive cardiomyopathy**, or HOCM (also called idiopathic hypertrophic subaortic stenosis, or IHSS). In this genetic disorder, disorganized proliferation of muscle fibers in the interventricular septum can cause significant septal hypertrophy. The resultant clinical repercussions can range from severe and life threatening to virtually none. Death can result from (1) obstruction to left ventricular outflow by the hypertrophied muscle; (2) impaired filling of the stiff, hypertrophied left ventricle during diastole; or (3) an abnormal ventricular rhythm (see the next chapter). The classic features on the resting EKG are the following:

1. Ventricular hypertrophy

2. Repolarization abnormalities in those leads with the tallest R waves

3. Q waves, of uncertain etiology, in the inferior and lateral leads.

Although this case was patently unfair, you may have recognized some of the features we have been talking about in this chapter, namely, the presence of criteria for left ventricular hypertrophy, especially in the precordial leads. Repolarization abnormalities are evident in all the left lateral leads (I, aVL, V5, and V6). Note, too, the deep Q waves in leads II, III, and aVF, typical of this disorder.

The timely intervention of his fellow runner saved Tom's life. It turned out that Tom had experienced similar, albeit less severe, episodes in the past, characterized by light-headedness and chest pain. He was subsequently advised to avoid strenuous and competitive exercise (mild to moderate aerobic activity is fine), and was placed on verapamil, a calcium-channel blocker, which prevented any recurrence of his symptoms. **Verapamil** reduces the strength of ventricular contraction, thereby decreasing the obstruction from the hypertrophied muscle, and improves the compliance of the stiffened ventricle. **Beta-blockers** are also used in this condition; they also lessen the risk for significant ischemia and may prevent arrhythmias. Placement of an implantable cardioverter-defibrillator (ICD) is also a strong consideration.

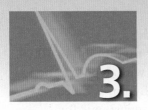

3. Arrhythmias

In this chapter you will learn:

1 | what an arrhythmia is, and what it does (and doesn't) do to people

2 | about rhythm strips, Holter monitors, and event monitors

3 | how to determine the heart rate from the EKG

4 | the five basic types of arrhythmias

5 | how to recognize the four common sinus arrhythmias

6 | what an ectopic rhythm is, and the mechanisms of its formation

7 | to ask The Four Questions that will let you recognize and diagnose the common ectopic arrhythmias that originate in the atria, the atrioventricular (AV) node, and the ventricles

8 | how to distinguish supraventricular arrhythmias from ventricular arrhythmias, both clinically and on the EKG

9 | how Programmed Electrical Stimulation and other techniques have revolutionized the diagnosis and treatment of certain arrhythmias

10 | about the cases of Lola deB., George M., and Frederick vanZ., which will leave you feeling astonished by how easily you have mastered material that has cowed the high and mighty.

The resting heart normally beats with a regular rhythm, 60 to 100 times per minute. Because each beat originates with depolarization of the sinus node, the usual, everyday cardiac rhythm is called *normal sinus rhythm*. Anything else is called an *arrhythmia* (or, more accurately, a *dysrhythmia*, but let's stick to the conventional terminology in the discussion to follow). The term *arrhythmia* refers to any disturbance in the rate, regularity, site of origin, or conduction of the cardiac electrical impulse. An arrhythmia can be a single aberrant beat (or even a prolonged pause between beats) or a sustained rhythm disturbance that can persist for the lifetime of the patient.

Not every arrhythmia is abnormal or dangerous. For example, heart rates as low as 35 to 40 beats per minute are common and quite normal in well-trained athletes. Single abnormal beats, originating elsewhere in the heart than the sinus node, frequently occur in the majority of healthy individuals.

Many arrhythmias, however, can be dangerous, and some require immediate therapy to prevent sudden death. The diagnosis of an arrhythmia is one of the most important things an EKG can do, and nothing yet has been found that can do it better.

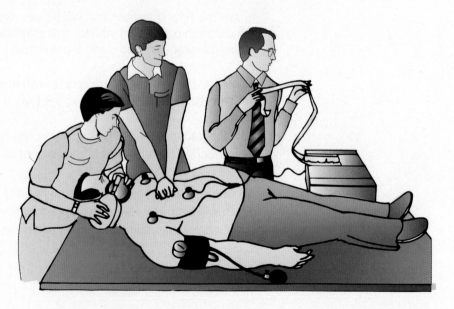

The Clinical Manifestations of Arrhythmias

When should you suspect that someone had or is having an arrhythmia?

Many arrhythmias go unnoticed by the patient and are picked up incidentally on a routine physical examination or EKG. Frequently, however, arrhythmias elicit one of several characteristic symptoms.

First and foremost are *palpitations*, an awareness of one's own heartbeat. Patients may describe intermittent accelerations or decelerations of their heartbeat, or a sustained rapid heartbeat that may be regular or irregular. The sensation may be no more than a mild nuisance or a truly terrifying experience.

More serious are symptoms of decreased cardiac output, which can occur when the arrhythmia compromises cardiac function. Among these are *light-headedness* and *syncope* (a sudden faint).

Rapid arrhythmias can increase the oxygen demands of the myocardium and cause *angina* (chest pain). The sudden onset of an arrhythmia in a patient with underlying cardiac disease can also precipitate *congestive heart failure*.

Sometimes, the first clinical manifestation of an arrhythmia is *sudden death*. Patients in the throes of an acute myocardial infarction are at a greatly increased risk for arrhythmic sudden death, which is why they are hospitalized in cardiac care units (CCUs) where their heart rate and rhythm can be continuously monitored.

Increasingly, the EKG has become helpful in identifying conditions that *predispose* to malignant arrhythmias and sudden death and thereby allow the initiation of lifesaving intervention *before* the catastrophic event. These conditions can be inherited or acquired. Most common among these are repolarization abnormalities that prolong the QT interval, a dangerous substrate for potentially lethal arrhythmias (more on this later).

Why Arrhythmias Happen

It is often impossible to identify the underlying cause of an arrhythmia, but a careful search for treatable precipitating factors must always be made. The mnemonic, HIS DEBS, should help you remember those arrhythmogenic factors that should be considered whenever you encounter a patient with an arrhythmia.

H—Hypoxia: A myocardium deprived of oxygen is an irritable myocardium. Pulmonary disorders, whether severe chronic lung disease or an acute pulmonary embolus, are major precipitants of cardiac arrhythmias.

I—Ischemia and Irritability: We have already mentioned that myocardial infarctions are a common setting for arrhythmias. Angina, even without the actual death of myocardial cells associated with infarction, is also a major precipitant. Occasionally, myocarditis, an inflammation of the heart muscle often caused by routine viral infections, can induce an arrhythmia.

S—Sympathetic Stimulation: Enhanced sympathetic tone from any cause (*e.g.*, hyperthyroidism, congestive heart failure, nervousness, exercise) can elicit arrhythmias.

D—Drugs: Many drugs can cause arrhythmias. Ironically, the antiarrhythmic drugs themselves, such as quinidine, are among the leading culprits.

E—Electrolyte Disturbances: Hypokalemia is notorious for its ability to induce arrhythmias, but imbalances of calcium and magnesium can also be responsible.

B—Bradycardia: A very slow heart rate seems to predispose to arrhythmias. One could include the bradytachycardia syndrome (also called the sick sinus syndrome) in this category.

S—Stretch: Enlargement and hypertrophy of the atria and ventricles can produce arrhythmias. This is one way in which congestive heart failure and valvular disease can cause arrhythmias.

Rhythm Strips

In order to identify an arrhythmia correctly, it is often necessary to view the heart rhythm over a much longer period of time than the few complexes present on the standard 12-lead EKG. When an arrhythmia is suspected, either clinically or electrocardiographically, it is standard practice to run a *rhythm strip*, a long tracing of a single lead or multiple leads. Any lead can be chosen, but it obviously makes sense to choose the lead that provides you with the most information. The rhythm strip makes it much easier to identify any irregularities or intermittent bursts of unusual electrical activity.

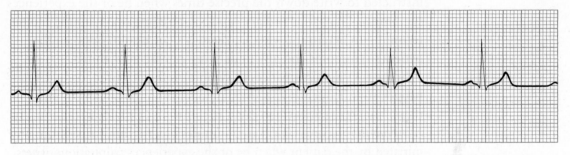

A typical rhythm strip. It can be as short or as long as you need to decipher the rhythm. This particular strip represents a continuous recording of lead II in a patient with normal sinus rhythm, the normal rhythm of the heart.

Holter Monitors and Event Monitors

The ultimate rhythm strip is provided by the *Holter monitor*, or *ambulatory monitor*. The Holter monitor is essentially a portable EKG machine with a memory. The patient wears it for 24 to 48 hours, and a complete record of the patient's heart rhythm is stored and later analyzed for any arrhythmic activity. The monitor can employ one or, more often, two leads (one precordial lead and one limb lead).

Holter monitoring is especially valuable when the suspected arrhythmia is an infrequent occurrence and is therefore unlikely to be captured on a random 12-lead EKG. Clearly, the longer one can monitor the patient, the better the chance that the arrhythmia will be detected. Further information can be obtained if the patient is instructed to write down the precise times when he or she experiences symptoms. The patient's diary can then be compared with the Holter recording to determine whether there is a correlation between the patient's symptoms and any underlying cardiac arrhythmia.

Some rhythm disturbances or symptoms suspicious for arrhythmias happen so infrequently that even a Holter monitor is likely to miss them. For these patients, an event monitor may provide a solution. An *event monitor* records only 3 to 5 minutes of a rhythm strip, but it is initiated by the patient when he or she experiences palpitations. The resultant EKG recording is sent out over the phone lines for evaluation. In this manner, multiple recordings can be made over the course of the several months during which the patient has rented the monitor.

Still other abnormal rhythms are so short-lived or infrequent that they are missed by any standard type of patient-activated mechanism. Two technologies are available for use in this situation. The first is a cell phone–based monitor that provides hospital-level telemetry in the ambulatory setting at home for up to 4 weeks. The second is a surgically implanted event recorder that is inserted under the skin of the patient with a small (1-inch) incision. These event recorders can be safely left in place for over a year and can automatically record and store in their memory rapid or slow heart rates (the rates that trigger the recorder are programmable). The patient can also activate the recorder whenever symptoms occur. The recorded data can be easily downloaded, typically every few months, by telemetry communication.

12.5 mm/sec, 25.0 mm/mV   ▲ = Activation point

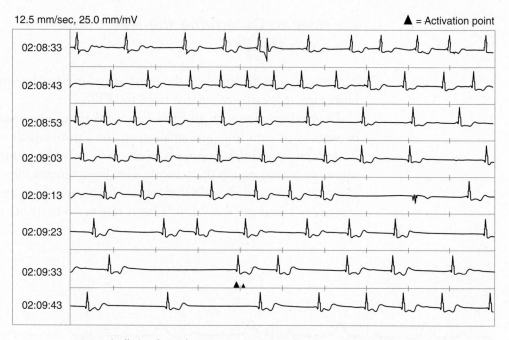

A surgically implanted event monitor recording in a patient with syncope. The small vertical dashes mark off intervals of 1 second. The 3-second pause near the bottom of the strip activates the monitor, which then stores the EKG tracing from several minutes before to several minutes after the activation point. The stored recording is then downloaded and printed at a later time. In this patient, the long pause was associated with a near-syncopal episode.

How to Determine the Heart Rate From the EKG

The first step in determining the heart's rhythm is to determine the heart rate. It is easily calculated from the EKG.

The horizontal axis on an EKG represents time. The distance between each light line (one small square or 1 mm) equals 0.04 seconds, and the distance between each heavy line (one large square or 5 mm) equals 0.2 seconds. Five large squares therefore constitute 1 second. A cycle that repeats itself every five large squares represents 1 beat per second, or a heart rate of 60 beats per minute.

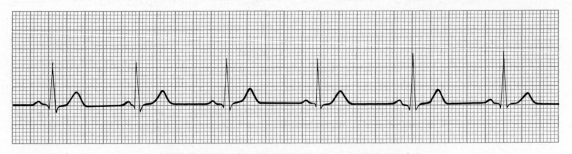

Every QRS complex is separated by five large squares (1 second). A rhythm occurring once every second occurs 60 times every minute.

A Simple Three-Step Method for Calculating the Heart Rate

1. Find an R wave that falls on, or nearly on, one of the heavy lines.

2. Count the number of large squares until the next R wave.

3. Determine the rate in beats per minute as follows:

   - If there is one large square between successive R waves, then each R wave is separated by 0.2 seconds. Therefore, over the course of 1 full second, there will be 5 cycles of cardiac activity (1 second divided by 0.2 seconds), and over 1 minute, 300 cycles (5 × 60 seconds). The heart rate is therefore 300 beats per minute.

   - If there are two large squares between successive R waves, then each R wave is separated by 0.4 seconds. Therefore, over the course of 1 full second, there will be 2.5 cycles of cardiac activity (1 second divided by 0.4 seconds), and over 1 minute, 150 cycles (2.5 × 60 seconds). The heart rate is therefore 150 beats per minute.

By similar logic:

- Three large squares = 100 beats per minute

- Four large squares = 75 beats per minute

- Five large squares = 60 beats per minute

- Six large squares = 50 beats per minute

Notice that you can get the same answers by dividing 300 by the number of large squares between R waves (*e.g.*, 300 divided by 4 squares = 75). Even greater accuracy can be achieved by counting the total number *of small* squares between R waves and dividing 1,500 by this total.

What is the heart rate of the following strips?

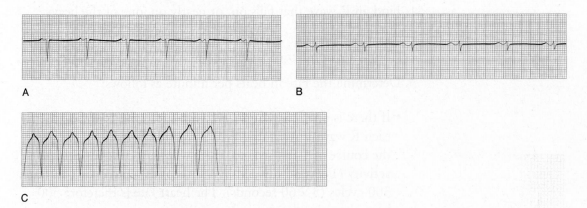

A   B

C

(*A*) About 75 beats per minute; (*B*) about 60 beats per minute;
(*C*) about 150 beats per minute.

If the second R wave falls *between* heavy lines, you can estimate
that the rate falls between the two extremes on either side.
What is the rate of the following strip?

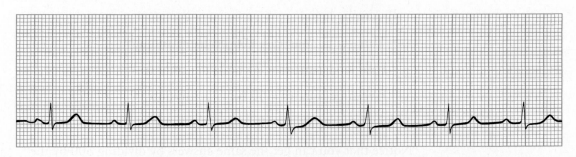

The R waves are slightly more than four squares apart—let's say four and
one-quarter. The rate must therefore be between 60 and 75 beats per
minute. If you guess 70, you'll be close. Alternatively, divide 300 by four and
one-quarter and get 70.6 beats per minute.

If the heart rate is very slow, you can still use this system; simply divide 300 by the number of large squares between complexes to get your answer. However, there is another method that some prefer. Every EKG strip is marked at 3-second intervals, usually with a series of little lines (or slashes or dots) at the top or bottom of the strip. Count the number of cycles within two of these intervals (6 seconds) and multiply by 10 (10 × 6 seconds = 60 seconds) to get the heart rate in beats per minute. Try it both ways on the example below:

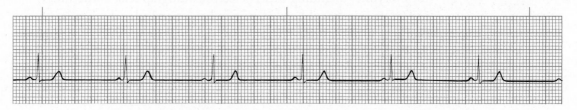

There are about five and one-half cycles within two of the 3-second intervals. The rate is therefore about 55 beats per minute.

The Five Basic Types of Arrhythmias

Of all of the subjects in electrocardiography, none is guaranteed to cause more anxiety (and palpitations) than the study of arrhythmias. There is no reason for this. First, once you have learned to recognize the basic patterns, nothing is easier than recognizing a classic arrhythmia. Second, the difficult arrhythmias are difficult for everyone, including expert electrocardiographers. Sometimes, in fact, it is impossible to identify what a particular rhythm is. Nothing gladdens one's heart more than the sight of two venerable cardiologists going at it over an insoluble rhythm disturbance.

The heart is capable of only five basic types of rhythm disturbances:

1. The electrical activity follows the usual conduction pathways we have already outlined, but it is either too fast, too slow, or irregular. These are *arrhythmias of sinus origin*.

2. The electrical activity originates from a focus other than the sinus node. These are called *ectopic rhythms*.

3. The electrical activity is trapped within an electrical racetrack whose shape and boundaries are determined by various anatomic or electrical myocardial features. These are called *reentrant arrhythmias*. They can occur anywhere in the heart.

4. The electrical activity originates in the sinus node and follows the usual pathways but encounters unexpected blocks and delays. These *conduction blocks* are discussed in Chapter 4.

5. The electrical activity follows accessory conduction pathways that bypass the normal ones, providing an electrical shortcut, or short circuit. These arrhythmias are termed *preexcitation syndromes*, and they are discussed in Chapter 5.

Arrhythmias of Sinus Origin

Sinus Tachycardia and Sinus Bradycardia

Normal sinus rhythm is the normal rhythm of the heart. Depolarization originates spontaneously within the sinus node. The rate is regular and between 60 and 100 beats per minute. If the rhythm speeds up beyond 100, it is called *sinus tachycardia;* if it slows down below 60, it is called *sinus bradycardia.*

Sinus tachycardia and sinus bradycardia can be normal or pathologic. Strenuous exercise, for example, can accelerate the heart rate well over 100 beats per minute, whereas resting heart rates below 60 beats per minute are typical in well-conditioned athletes. On the other hand, alterations in the rate at which the sinus node fires can accompany significant heart disease. Sinus tachycardia can occur in patients with congestive heart failure or severe lung disease, or it can be the only presenting sign of hyperthyroidism. Sinus bradycardia is the most common rhythm disturbance seen in the early stages of an acute myocardial infarction; in otherwise healthy individuals, it can result from enhanced vagal tone and cause fainting.

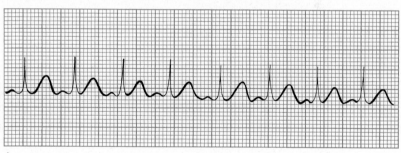

A

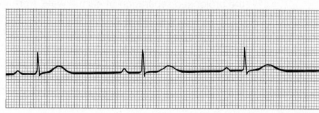

B

(*A*) Sinus tachycardia. Each beat is separated by two and one-half large squares for a rate of 120 beats per minute. (*B*) Sinus bradycardia. More than seven large squares separate each beat, and the rate is 40 to 45 beats per minute.

Sinus Arrhythmia

Often, the EKG will reveal a rhythm that appears in all respects to be normal sinus rhythm except that it is slightly irregular. This is called *sinus arrhythmia*. Most often, it is a normal phenomenon, reflecting the variation in heart rate that accompanies inspiration and expiration. Inspiration accelerates the heart rate, and expiration slows it down.

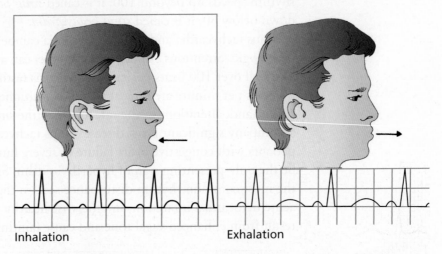

Inhalation   Exhalation

Sinus arrhythmia. The heart rate accelerates with inspiration and slows with expiration.

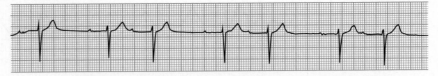

A beautiful example of sinus arrhythmia. You may have also noticed the prolonged separation of each P wave from its ensuing QRS complex (*i.e.*, a prolonged PR interval). This represents a conduction delay called first-degree atrioventricular (AV) block; it is discussed in Chapter 4.

Sinus Arrest, Asystole, and Escape Beats

Sinus arrest occurs when the sinus node stops firing. If nothing else were to happen, the EKG would show a flat line without any electrical activity, and the patient would die. Prolonged electrical inactivity is called *asystole*.

Fortunately, virtually all myocardial cells have the ability to behave as pacemakers. Ordinarily, the fastest pacemaker drives the heart, and under normal circumstances, the fastest pacemaker is the sinus node. The sinus node *overdrives* the other pacemaker cells by delivering its wave of depolarization throughout the myocardium before its potential competitors can complete their own, more leisurely, spontaneous depolarization. With sinus arrest, however, these other pacemakers can spring into action in a kind of rescue mission. These rescuing beats, originating outside the sinus node, are called *escape beats*.

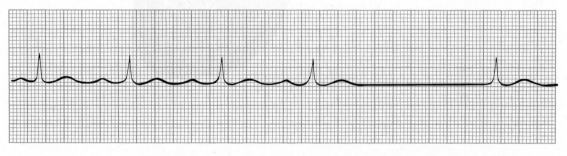

Sinus arrest occurs after the fourth beat. The fifth beat, restoring electrical activity to the heart, is a junctional escape beat (see the next page for further explanation). Note the absence of a P wave before this last beat.

Nonsinus Pacemakers

Like the sinus node, which typically fires between 60 and 100 times each minute, the other potential pacemaker cells of the heart have their own intrinsic rhythm. *Atrial pacemakers* usually discharge at a rate of 60 to 75 beats per minute. Pacemaker cells located near the AV node, called *junctional pacemakers*, typically discharge at 40 to 60 beats per minute. *Ventricular pacemaker* cells usually discharge at 30 to 45 beats per minute.

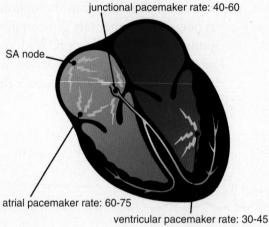

junctional pacemaker rate: 40-60

SA node

atrial pacemaker rate: 60-75

ventricular pacemaker rate: 30-45

Each of these nonsinus pacemakers can rescue an inadequate sinus node by providing just one or a continual series of escape beats. Of all of the available escape mechanisms, *junctional escape* is by far the most common.

With junctional escape, depolarization originates near the AV node, and the usual pattern of atrial depolarization does not occur. As a result, a normal P wave is not seen. Most often, there is no P wave at all. Occasionally, however, a retrograde P wave may be seen, representing atrial depolarization moving *backward* from the AV node into the atria. The mean electrical axis of this *retrograde P wave* is reversed 180° from that of the normal P wave. Thus, whereas the normal P wave is upright in lead II and inverted in lead AVR, the retrograde P wave is inverted in lead II and upright in lead AVR.

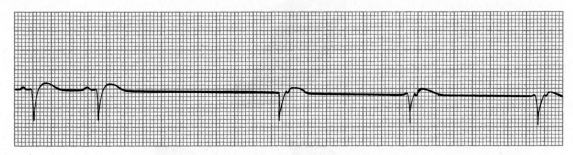

Junctional escape. The first two beats are normal sinus beats with a normal P wave preceding each QRS complex. There is then a long pause followed by a series of three junctional escape beats occurring at a rate of 40 to 45 beats per minute. Retrograde P waves can be seen buried in the early portion of the T waves. Retrograde P waves can occur before, after, or during the QRS complex, depending on the relative timing of atrial and ventricular depolarization. If atrial and ventricular depolarization occur simultaneously, the much larger QRS complexes will mask the retrograde P waves.

Sinus Arrest Versus Sinus Exit Block

Because sinus node depolarization is *not* recorded on the EKG, it is impossible to determine whether a prolonged sinus pause is due to sinus arrest or to failure of the sinus depolarization to be transmitted out of the node and into the atria, a situation called *sinus exit block*. You may hear these different terms bandied about from time to time, but for all intents and purposes, sinus arrest and sinus exit block mean the same thing: there is a failure of the sinus mechanism to deliver its current into the surrounding tissue.

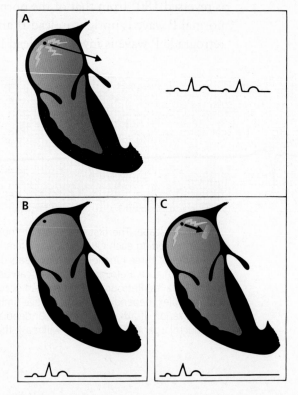

(*A*) Normal sinus rhythm. The sinus node fires repeatedly, and waves of depolarization spread out into the atria. (*B*) Sinus arrest. The sinus node falls silent. No current is generated, and the EKG shows no electrical activity. (*C*) Sinus exit block. The sinus node continues to fire, but the wave of depolarization fails to exit the sinus node into the atrial myocardium. Again, the EKG shows no electrical activity; there is not sufficient voltage to generate a detectable P wave.

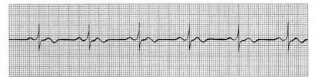

Normal sinus rhythm

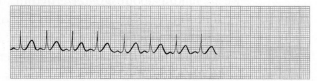

Sinus tachycardia

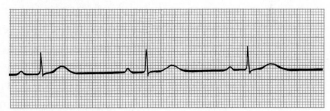

Sinus bradycardia

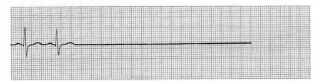

Sinus arrest or exit block

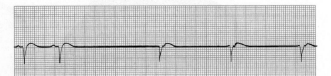

Sinus arrest or exit block with junctional escape

Special note for the electrically infatuated: there is a way in which transient sinus arrest and sinus exit block can sometimes be distinguished on the EKG. With sinus arrest, resumption of sinus electrical activity occurs at any random time (the sinus node simply resumes firing). However, with sinus exit block, the sinus node has continued to fire silently, so when the block is lifted, the sinus node resumes depolarizing the atria after a pause that is some integer multiple of the normal cycle (exactly one missed P wave, or exactly two missed P waves, or more).

Ectopic Rhythms

Ectopic rhythms are abnormal rhythms that arise from elsewhere than the sinus node. In this way, they resemble escape beats, but here we are talking about *sustained* rhythms, not just one or a few beats. Ectopic rhythms can be caused by any of the precipitating factors described previously.

At the cellular level, they arise from enhanced automaticity of a nonsinus node site, either a single focus or a roving one. As we have already stressed, the fastest pacemaker usually drives the heart, and under normal circumstances, the fastest pacemaker is the sinus node. Under abnormal circumstances, however, any of the other pacemakers scattered throughout the heart can be accelerated, that is, stimulated to depolarize faster and faster until they can overdrive the normal sinus mechanism and establish their own transient or sustained ectopic rhythm. Among the most common causes of enhanced automaticity are digitalis toxicity and beta-adrenergic stimulation from inhaler therapies used to treat asthma and chronic obstructive lung disease. We will see examples of ectopic rhythms in the pages to come.

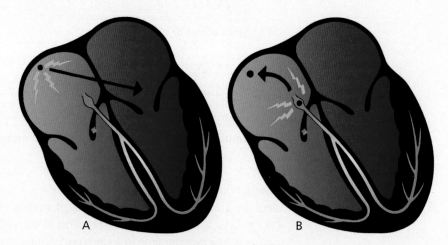

(*A*) Normally, the sinus node drives the heart. (*B*) If another potential pacemaker (*e.g.*, the AV junction) is accelerated, it can take over the heart and overdrive the sinus node.

Reentrant Rhythms

The second major cause of nonsinus arrhythmias is called *reentry*. Whereas enhanced automaticity represents a disorder of *impulse formation* (*i.e.*, new impulses formed elsewhere than the sinus node take over the heart), reentry represents a disorder of *impulse transmission*. The results, however, are similar: creation of a focus of abnormal electrical activity. Here is how reentry works:

Picture a wave of depolarization arriving at two adjacent regions of myocardium, *A* and *B*, as shown in part *1* of the figure on the next page. *A* and *B* conduct the current at the same rate, and the wave of depolarization rushes past, unperturbed, on its way to new destinations. This is the way things usually operate.

Suppose, however, that pathway *B* transmits the wave of depolarization more slowly than does pathway *A*. This can result, for example, if pathway *B* has been damaged by ischemic disease or fibrosis, or if the two pathways are receiving different degrees of input from the autonomic nervous system. This situation is depicted in part *2* of the figure. The wave of depolarization now rushes through pathway *A* but is held up in pathway *B*. The impulse emerging from pathway *A* can now return back through pathway *B*, setting up an uninterrupted revolving circuit along the two pathways (see figure, part *3*). As the electrical impulse spins in this loop, waves of depolarization are sent out in all directions. This is called a *reentry loop*, and it behaves like an electrical racetrack, providing a source of electrical activation that can overdrive the sinus mechanism and run the heart.

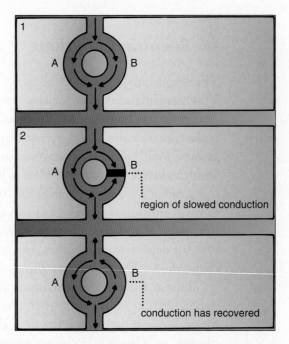

A model showing how a reentrant circuit becomes established.
(*1*) Normally, pathways *A* and *B* (any two adjacent regions of cardiac function) conduct current equally well. (*2*) Here, however, conduction through pathway *B* is temporarily slowed. Current passing down *A* can then turn back and conduct in a retrograde fashion through *B*. (*3*) The reentry loop is established.

A reentry loop can vary greatly in size. It can be limited to a small loop within a single anatomic site (*e.g.,* the AV node), it can loop through an entire chamber (either an atrium or ventricle), or it can even involve both an atrium and ventricle if there is an accessory pathway of conduction connecting the two chambers (this last point is made more obvious in Chapter 5).

The Four Questions

As you will see in just a moment, all of the clinically important nonsinus arrhythmias—the ones you have probably heard of—are either ectopic or reentrant in origin. It is therefore critical to be able to identify them, and you will spend the rest of this chapter learning exactly how to do that. This may sound like a tall order, but to assess any rhythm disturbance on the EKG you only need to answer four questions:

Are Normal P Waves Present? The emphasis here is on the word *normal*. If the answer is yes, if there are *normal*-appearing P waves with a *normal* P wave axis, then the origin of the arrhythmia is almost certainly within the atria. If no P waves are present, then the rhythm must have originated below the atria, in the AV node or the ventricles. The presence of P waves with an *abnormal* axis may reflect retrograde activation of the atria from impulses originating below the sinus node from some other atrial focus or in the AV node or in the ventricles, that is, from current flowing backward into the atria through the AV node or through an accessory pathway (more on all of this later). An abnormal P wave axis does not guarantee that the origin of the rhythm is located below the atria, whereas a normal P wave axis is pretty good assurance that the rhythm originates above the AV node.

Are the QRS Complexes Narrow (Less Than 0.12 Seconds in Duration) or Wide (Greater Than 0.12 Seconds in Duration)? A narrow normal QRS complex implies that ventricular depolarization is proceeding along the usual pathways (AV node to His bundle to bundle branches to Purkinje cells). This is the most efficient means of conduction, requiring the least amount of time, so the resulting QRS complex is of short duration (narrow). A narrow QRS complex, therefore, indicates that the origin of the rhythm must be at or above the AV node. A wide QRS complex usually implies that the origin of ventricular depolarization is within the ventricles themselves. Depolarization is initiated within the ventricular myocardium, not the conduction system, and therefore spreads much more slowly. Conduction does *not* follow the most efficient pathway, and the QRS complex is of long duration (wide).

(The distinction between wide and narrow QRS complexes, although very useful, cannot, unfortunately, be fully relied on to assess the origin of an arrhythmia. We'll see why shortly.)

Questions 1 and 2 thus help to make the important distinction of whether an arrhythmia is ventricular or supraventricular (atrial or junctional) in origin.

What Is the Relationship Between the P Waves and the QRS Complexes? If the P wave and QRS complexes correlate in the usual one-to-one fashion, with a single P wave preceding each QRS complex, then the rhythm almost certainly has a sinus or other atrial origin. Sometimes, however, the atria and ventricles depolarize and contract independently of each other. This will be manifested on the EKG by a lack of correlation between the P waves and QRS complexes, a situation termed *AV dissociation*.

Is the Rhythm Regular or Irregular? This is often the most immediately obvious characteristic of a particular rhythm and is sometimes the most critical.

Whenever you look at an EKG, you will need to assess the rhythm. These four questions should become an intrinsic part of your thinking:

1. Are normal P waves present?

2. Are the QRS complexes narrow or wide?

3. What is the relationship between the P waves and the QRS complexes?

4. Is the rhythm regular or irregular?

For the normal EKG (normal sinus rhythm), the answers are easy:

1. Yes, there are normal P waves.

2. The QRS complexes are narrow.

3. There is one P wave for every QRS complex.

4. The rhythm is essentially regular.

We will now see what happens when the answers are different.

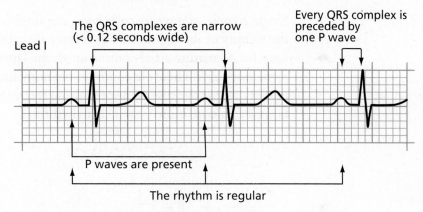

Normal sinus rhythm and "The Four Questions" answered.

Supraventricular Arrhythmias

Let us look first at the arrhythmias that originate in the atria or the AV node, the **supraventricular arrhythmias.**

Atrial arrhythmias can consist of a single beat or a sustained rhythm disturbance lasting for a few seconds or many years.

Atrial and Junctional Premature Beats

Single ectopic supraventricular beats can originate in the atria or in the vicinity of the AV node. The former are called *atrial premature beats* (or premature atrial contractions); the latter, *junctional premature beats*. These are common phenomena, neither indicating underlying cardiac disease nor requiring treatment. They can, however, initiate more sustained arrhythmias.

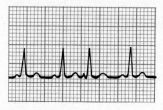

A

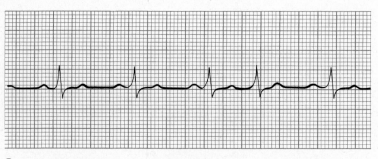

B

(*A*) The third beat is an atrial premature beat. Note how the P wave contour of the premature beat differs from that of the normal sinus beat. (*B*) The fourth beat is a junctional premature beat. There is no P wave preceding the premature QRS complex.

An atrial premature beat can be distinguished from a normal sinus beat by the *contour* of the P wave and by the timing of the beat.

Contour. Because an atrial premature beat originates at an atrial site distant from the sinus node, atrial depolarization does not occur in the usual manner, and the configuration of the resultant P wave differs from that of the sinus P waves. If the site of origin of the atrial premature beat is far from the sinus node, the axis of the atrial premature beat will also differ from that of the normal P waves.

Timing. An atrial premature beat comes too early; that is, it intrudes itself before the next anticipated sinus wave.

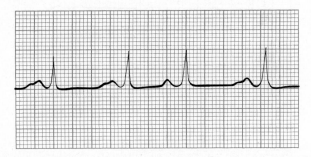

The third beat is an atrial premature beat. The P wave is shaped differently from the other, somewhat unusual-looking P waves, and the beat is clearly premature.

With junctional premature beats, there is usually no visible P wave, but sometimes a retrograde P wave may be seen. This is just like the case with the junctional escape beats seen with sinus arrest.

What is the difference between a junctional *premature* beat and a junctional *escape* beat? They look exactly alike, but the junctional premature beat occurs *early*, prematurely, interposing itself into the normal sinus rhythm. An escape beat occurs *late*, following a pause when the sinus node has failed to fire.

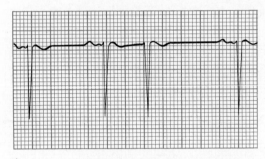

A

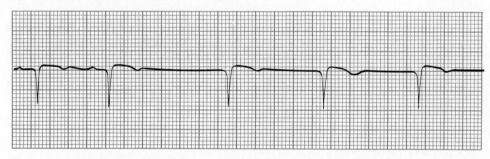

B

(*A*) A junctional premature beat. The third beat is obviously premature, and there is no P wave preceding the QRS complex. (*B*) The third beat is a junctional escape beat, establishing a sustained junctional rhythm. It looks just like a junctional premature beat, but it occurs late, following a prolonged pause, rather than prematurely.

Both atrial and junctional premature beats are usually conducted normally to the ventricles, and the resultant QRS complex is therefore narrow.

Sometimes an atrial premature beat may occur sufficiently early that the AV node will not have recovered (i.e., repolarized) from the previous conducted beat and will therefore be unable to conduct the atrial premature beat into the ventricles. The ECG may then show only a P wave without an ensuing QRS complex. This beat is then termed a *blocked atrial premature contraction.*

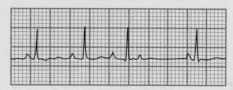

The fourth P wave is a blocked PAC.

There are five types of *sustained* supraventricular arrhythmias that you must learn to recognize:

1. Paroxysmal supraventricular tachycardia (PSVT), sometimes also called AV nodal reentrant tachycardia

2. Atrial flutter

3. Atrial fibrillation

4. Multifocal atrial tachycardia (MAT)

5. Paroxysmal atrial tachycardia (PAT), sometimes also called ectopic atrial tachycardia.

Paroxysmal Supraventricular Tachycardia

PSVT is a very common arrhythmia. Its onset is sudden, usually initiated by a premature supraventricular beat (atrial or junctional), and its termination is just as abrupt. It can occur in perfectly normal hearts; there may be no underlying cardiac disease at all. Persons with PSVT typically present with palpitations, shortness of breath, dizziness and—rarely—syncope. Not uncommonly, alcohol, coffee, or just sheer excitement can elicit this rhythm disturbance.

PSVT is an *absolutely regular rhythm*, with a rate usually between 150 and 250 beats per minute. There are several types of PSVT. The most common type is driven by a reentrant circuit looping within the AV node (hence it is often referred to as AV *nodal reentrant tachycardia*). Retrograde P waves may sometimes be seen in leads II or III, but your best chance would be to look in lead V1 for what is called a pseudo-R', a little blip in the QRS complex that represents the superimposed retrograde P wave. More often than not, however, the P waves are so buried in the QRS complexes that they cannot be identified with any confidence. As with most supraventricular arrhythmias, the QRS complex is usually narrow.

Another type of PSVT occurs in patients with anomalous conduction pathways and is discussed in Chapter 5.

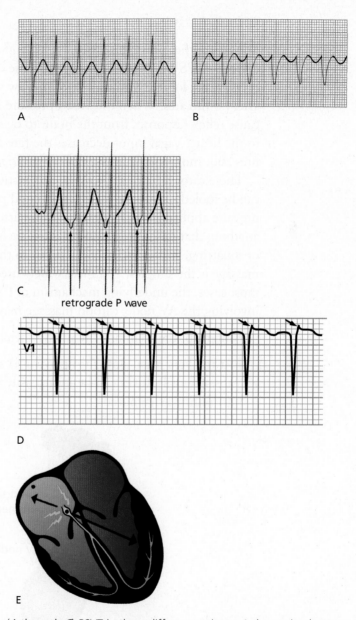

(*A* through *C*) PSVT in three different patients. *A* shows simultaneous activation of the atria and ventricles; therefore, the retrograde P waves are lost in the QRS complexes. *B* shows a supraventricular tachycardia mimicking a more serious rhythm called ventricular tachycardia (VT) (see page 138). In *C*, retrograde P waves can be seen. (*D*) A good example of the pseudo-R′ configuration in lead V1 representing the retrograde P waves (*arrows*) of PSVT. (*E*) The AV node is usually the site of the reentrant circuit that causes the arrhythmia. Atrial depolarization therefore occurs in reverse, and if P waves can be seen, their axis will be shifted nearly 180° from normal (retrograde P waves).

Carotid Massage

Massaging the carotid artery can help to *diagnose* and *terminate* an episode of PSVT. Baroreceptors that sense changes in the blood pressure are located at the angle of the jaw where the common carotid artery bifurcates. When the blood pressure rises, these baroreceptors cause reflex responses from the brain to be sent along the vagus nerve to the heart. Vagal input decreases the rate at which the sinus node fires and, more importantly, *slows conduction through the AV node.*

These carotid baroreceptors are not particularly shrewd, and they can be fooled into thinking that the blood pressure is rising by gentle pressure applied *externally* to the carotid artery. (For that matter, anything that raises the blood pressure, such as a Valsalva maneuver or squatting, will stimulate vagal input to the heart, but carotid massage is the simplest and most widely used maneuver.) Because, in most cases, the underlying mechanism of PSVT is a reentrant circuit involving the AV node, carotid massage may accomplish the following:

- Interrupt the reentrant circuit and thereby terminate the arrhythmia

- At the very least, slow the arrhythmia so that the presence or absence of P waves can be more easily determined and the arrhythmia diagnosed

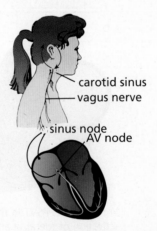

carotid sinus
vagus nerve
sinus node
AV node

The carotid sinus contains baroreceptors that influence vagal input to the heart, primarily affecting the sinus node and AV node. Stimulation of the right carotid baroreceptors primarily stimulates sinus node vagal input, whereas stimulation of the left carotid baroreceptors is more likely to affect the vagal input to the AV node.

How to Do Carotid Massage

Carotid massage must be done with great care.

1. Auscultate for carotid bruits. You do *not* want to cut off the last remaining trickle of blood to the brain nor dislodge an atherosclerotic plaque. If there is evidence of significant carotid disease, do *not* perform carotid massage.

2. With the patient lying flat, extend the neck and rotate the head slightly away from you.

3. Palpate the carotid artery at the angle of the jaw and apply gentle pressure for 10 to 15 seconds.

4. *Never* compress both carotid arteries simultaneously!

5. Try the right carotid first because the rate of success is somewhat better on this side. If it fails, however, go ahead and try the left carotid next.

6. Have a rhythm strip running during the entire procedure so that you can see what is happening. Always have equipment for resuscitation available; in rare instances, carotid massage may induce sinus arrest.

carotid massage begins

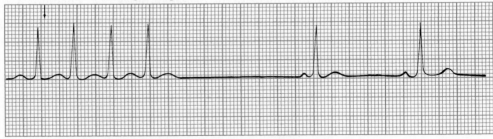

An episode of PSVT is broken almost at once by carotid massage. The new rhythm is a sinus bradycardia with a rate of 50 beats per minute.

For patients with an acute episode of PSVT that does not respond to carotid massage or other vagal maneuvers, pharmacologic intervention will usually terminate the arrhythmia. A bolus injection of adenosine, a short-acting AV nodal blocking agent, is almost always effective (avoid this drug in patients with bronchospastic lung disease). Second-line therapies include beta-blockers, calcium channel blockers, and—rarely—electrical cardioversion.

Atrial Flutter

Atrial flutter is less common than PSVT. It can occur in normal hearts or, more often, in patients with underlying cardiac pathology. The atrial activation in atrial flutter, as in PSVT, is absolutely regular but is even more rapid. P waves appear at a rate of 250 to 350 beats per minute. In its most common form, it is generated by a reentrant circuit that runs largely around the annulus of the tricuspid valve.

In atrial flutter, atrial depolarization occurs at such a rapid rate that discrete P waves separated by a flat baseline are not seen. Instead, the baseline continually rises and falls, producing so-called *flutter waves.* In some leads, usually leads II and III, these may be quite prominent and may create what has been termed a *saw-toothed pattern.*

The AV node cannot handle the extraordinary number of atrial impulses bombarding it—it simply doesn't have time to repolarize in time for each ensuing wave—and therefore, not all of the atrial impulses pass through the AV node to generate QRS complexes. Some just bump into a refractory node, and that is as far as they get. This phenomenon is called *AV block.* A 2:1 block is most common. This means that for every two visible flutter waves, one passes through the AV node to generate a QRS complex, and one does not. Blocks of 3:1 and 4:1 are also frequently seen. Carotid massage may increase the degree of block (*e.g.,* changing a 2:1 block to a 4:1 block), making it easier to identify the saw-toothed pattern. Because atrial flutter originates above the AV node, carotid massage will not result in termination of the rhythm.

carotid massage begins

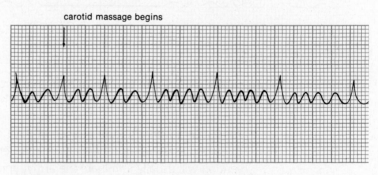

Atrial flutter. Carotid massage increases the block from 3:1 to 5:1.

The axis of the P waves (flutter waves) in atrial flutter depends upon whether the reentrant circuit rotates counterclockwise (the more common form, producing negative saw-tooth deflections in the inferior leads) or clockwise (positive deflections in the inferior leads) around the tricuspid valve.

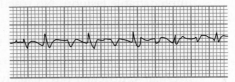

Atrial flutter. Lead II shows classic negative deflections.

Approximately 200,000 cases of atrial flutter are diagnosed each year in the United States. Common conditions associated with atrial flutter include the following:

Hypertension

Obesity

Diabetes mellitus

Electrolyte imbalances

Alcohol intoxication

Drug abuse, particularly cocaine and amphetamines

Pulmonary disease (e.g., chronic obstructive pulmonary disease and pulmonary embolism)

Thyrotoxicosis

Various underlying cardiac conditions, both congenital (*e.g.*, atrial septal defect) and acquired (*e.g.*, rheumatic valvular disease, coronary artery disease and congestive heart failure)

Although atrial flutter is rarely life threatening, the rapid ventricular response may cause shortness of breath or angina or precipitate or worsen congestive heart failure, which may mandate urgent clinical intervention. Electrical cardioversion is very effective at restoring normal sinus rhythm, although pharmacologic cardioversion is often first attempted in patients who are hemodynamically stable.

Atrial Fibrillation

In *atrial fibrillation*, atrial activity is completely chaotic, and the AV node may be bombarded with more than 500 impulses per minute! Whereas in atrial flutter a single constant reentrant circuit is responsible for the regular saw-toothed pattern on the EKG, in atrial fibrillation multiple reentrant circuits whirl around in totally unpredictable fashion. No true P waves can be seen. Instead, the baseline appears flat or undulates slightly. The AV node, faced with this extraordinary blitz of atrial impulses, allows only occasional impulses to pass through at variable intervals, generating an *irregularly irregular* ventricular rate, usually between 120 and 180 beats per minute. However, slower or faster ventricular responses (see figures *A* and *B* below) can often be seen.

This irregularly irregular appearance of QRS complexes in the absence of discrete P waves is the key to identifying atrial fibrillation. The wavelike forms that may often be seen on close inspection of the undulating baseline are called *fibrillation waves*.

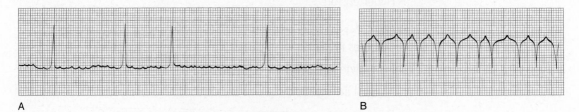

A   B

(*A*) Atrial fibrillation with a slow, irregular ventricular rate. (*B*) Another example of atrial fibrillation. In the absence of a clearly fibrillating baseline, the only clue that this rhythm is atrial fibrillation is the irregularly irregular appearance of the QRS complexes.

Carotid massage may slow the ventricular rate in atrial fibrillation, but it is rarely used in this setting because the diagnosis is usually obvious.

Atrial fibrillation is much more common than atrial flutter. It is the most common sustained arrhythmia in the general population, with an overall prevalence of up to 1.0% increasing with age so that it exceeds 8% among individuals over age 80. Underlying causes are similar to those for atrial flutter, with an especially high incidence of cardiac conditions, notably hypertensive heart disease, mitral valve disease, and coronary artery disease. Consideration of acute precipitants, such as pulmonary embolism, thyrotoxicosis, and pericarditis, must be stressed in the clinical evaluation of any patient with new-onset atrial fibrillation. An important cause of nocturnal episodes of atrial fibrillation is obstructive sleep apnea.

Symptoms of palpitations, chest pain, shortness of breath, and dizziness may occur, but a significant minority of patients experience no symptoms at all.

Restoration of normal sinus rhythm can be attempted through either electrical or pharmacologic cardioversion or ablative techniques (see following box and page 152), and is often temporarily successful. However, maintenance of normal sinus rhythm is often impossible to achieve, either because the arrhythmia is refractory to pharmacologic maintenance therapy or because of the many side effects associated with these agents.

Patients with persistent atrial fibrillation are at risk of systemic embolization. The fibrillating atria (often compared to a bag of worms) provide an excellent substrate for blood clots to form. Treatment of patients with an intermediate or high risk of stroke (*e.g.*, underlying hypertension, diabetes mellitus, mitral stenosis, or a prior history of transient ischemic event or stroke) must therefore include anticoagulation, traditionally with warfarin, but now more often with one of the new direct thrombin inhibitors, such as dabigatran. Whereas warfarin requires continual monitoring of the patient's prothrombin time (PT INR) to ensure adequate anticoagulation and to prevent overzealous anticoagulation with the attendant risk of a significant bleed, the direct thrombin inhibitors do not require continual monitoring and do not appear to be associated with any greater risk of bleeding complications.

Patients with persistent atrial fibrillation and a rapid ventricular response, particularly if associated with symptoms, may also require long-term pharmacologic therapy (*e.g.*, beta-blockers) to control their ventricular rate. For some, a so-called pill-in-the-pocket approach may be a useful adjunct to therapy, in which patients already on rate-control agents are instructed to take an additional pill whenever they feel the onset of symptoms.

Studies have shown little to no survival benefit of rhythm control versus rate control and anticoagulation. Rhythm control is generally attempted in younger patients, since restoration of normal sinus rhythm appears to improve perceived quality of life. In patients over 70, especially if asymptomatic, rate control with anticoagulation is a viable and often preferred alternative.

Recent work has suggested that somatic mutations in at least one gap-junction membrane protein involved in myocyte depolarization may account for some cases of atrial fibrillation previously considered idiopathic, and it is likely that other genetic mutations will be found. Additional evidence has strongly implicated ectopic beats occurring at the site where the pulmonary veins connect to the left atrium as instrumental in triggering atrial fibrillation in otherwise normal hearts. Thus, procedures utilizing catheter ablation aimed at this area have proven successful in preventing recurrent atrial fibrillation in some patients.

Multifocal Atrial Tachycardia and Wandering Atrial Pacemakers

MAT is an irregular rhythm occurring at a rate of 100 to 200 beats per minute. It probably results from the random firing of several different ectopic atrial foci. Sometimes, the rate is less than 100 beats per minute, in which case the arrhythmia is often called a *wandering atrial pacemaker.*

MAT is very common in patients with severe lung disease. It rarely requires treatment. Carotid massage has *no* effect on MAT. A wandering atrial pacemaker can be seen in normal, healthy hearts.

Like atrial fibrillation, MAT is an irregular rhythm. It can be distinguished from atrial fibrillation by the easily identifiable P waves occurring before each QRS complex. The P waves, originating from multiple sites in the atria, will vary in shape, and the interval between the different P waves and the QRS complexes will vary as well. In order to make the diagnosis of MAT, you need to identify at least three different P wave morphologies.

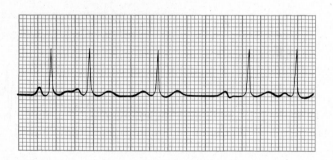

Multifocal atrial tachycardia. Note that (1) the P waves vary dramatically in shape; (2) the PR intervals vary; and (3) the ventricular rate is irregular.

In a wandering atrial pacemaker, at least three different P wave morphologies can be seen, but there will be at least two or three beats of each P wave morphology before the site moves on and creates the next morphology.

Paroxysmal Atrial Tachycardia

The last of our five supraventricular arrhythmias, *PAT*, is a regular rhythm with a rate of 100 to 200 beats per minute. It can result either from the enhanced automaticity of an ectopic atrial focus or from a reentrant circuit within the atria. The automatic type typically displays a warm-up period when it starts, during which the rhythm appears somewhat irregular, and a similar cool-down period when it terminates. The less common reentrant form starts abruptly with an atrial premature beat; this form of PAT has also been termed *atypical atrial flutter*.

PAT is most commonly seen in otherwise normal hearts. It can also be caused by digitalis toxicity.

How can you tell PAT from PSVT? Many times you can't. However, if you see a warm-up or cool-down period on the EKG, the rhythm is likely to be PAT. In addition, carotid massage can be very helpful: carotid massage will slow or terminate PSVT, whereas it has virtually no effect on PAT (other than some mild slowing).

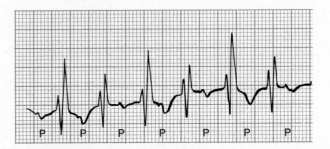

PAT. P waves are not always visible, but here they can be seen fairly easily. You may also notice the varying distance between the P waves and the ensuing QRS complexes; this reflects a varying conduction delay between the atria and ventricles that often accompanies PAT (but we are getting way ahead of ourselves; conduction delays are discussed in Chapter 4).

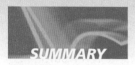

SUMMARY — Supraventricular Arrhythmias

Arrhythmia	Characteristics	EKG
PSVT	Regular P waves are retrograde if visible Rate: 150–250 bpm Carotid massage: slows or terminates	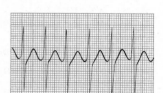
Flutter	Regular, saw-toothed 2:1, 3:1, 4:1, etc., block Atrial rate: 250–350 bpm Ventricular rate: one-half, one-third, one-quarter, etc., of atrial rate Carotid massage: increases block	carotid massage begins 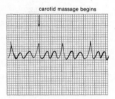
Fibrillation	Irregular Undulating baseline Atrial rate: 350–500 bpm Ventricular rate: variable Carotid massage: may slow ventricular rate	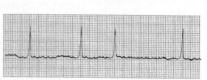
MAT	Irregular At least three different P wave morphologies Rate: 100–200 bpm; sometimes less than 100 bpm Carotid massage: no effect	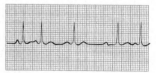
PAT	Regular Rate: 100–200 bpm Characteristic warm-up period in the automatic form Carotid massage: no effect, or only mild slowing	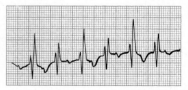

Ventricular Arrhythmias

Ventricular arrhythmias are rhythm disturbances arising below the AV node.

Premature Ventricular Contractions

Premature ventricular contractions (PVCs), are certainly the most common of the ventricular arrhythmias. **The QRS complex of a PVC appears wide and bizarre** because ventricular depolarization does not follow the normal conduction pathways. However, the QRS complex may not appear wide in all leads, so scan the entire 12-lead EKG before making your diagnosis. The QRS duration must be at least 0.12 seconds in most leads to make the diagnosis of a PVC. A retrograde P wave may sometimes be seen, but it is more common to see no P wave at all. A PVC is usually followed by a prolonged compensatory pause before the next beat appears. Less commonly, a PVC may occur between two normally conducted beats without a compensatory pause. These are called *interpolated PVCs*.

Isolated PVCs are common in normal hearts and rarely require treatment. An isolated PVC in the setting of an acute myocardial infarction, however, is more ominous because it can trigger ventricular tachycardia (VT) or ventricular fibrillation, both of which are life-threatening arrhythmias.

PVCs typically occur randomly, but they may alternate with normal sinus beats in a regular pattern. If the ratio is one normal sinus beat to one PVC, the rhythm is called *bigeminy*. *Trigeminy* refers to two normal sinus beats for every one PVC, and so on.

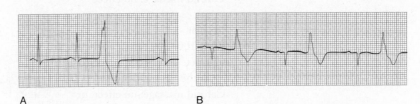

A   B

(*A*) A PVC. Note the compensatory pause before the next beat.
(*B*) Bigeminy. PVCs and sinus beats alternate in a 1:1 fashion.

When should you worry about PVCs? Certain situations have been identified in which PVCs appear to pose an increased risk for triggering VT, ventricular fibrillation, and death. These situations are summarized in *the rules of malignancy:*

1. Frequent PVCs

2. Runs of consecutive PVCs, especially three or more in a row

3. Multiform PVCs, in which the PVCs vary in their site of origin and hence in their appearance

4. PVCs falling on the T wave of the previous beat, called the "R-on-T" phenomenon. The T wave is a vulnerable period in the cardiac cycle, and a PVC falling there is more likely to set off VT.

5. Any PVC occurring in the setting of an acute myocardial infarction

Although PVCs meeting one or several of these criteria are associated with an increased risk for developing a life-threatening arrhythmia, there is no evidence that suppressing these PVCs with antiarrhythmic medication reduces mortality in any setting.

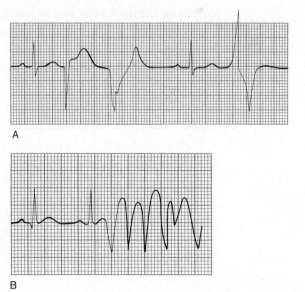

(*A*) Beats 1 and 4 are sinus in origin. The other three beats are PVCs. The PVCs differ from each other in shape (multiform), and two occur in a row. (*B*) A PVC falls on the T wave of the second sinus beat, initiating a run of VT.

Ventricular Tachycardia

A run of three or more consecutive PVCs is called *ventricular tachycardia* (VT). The rate is usually between 120 and 200 beats per minute and, unlike PSVT, may be slightly irregular (although it may take a very fine eye to see this). Sustained VT is an emergency, presaging cardiac arrest and requiring immediate treatment.

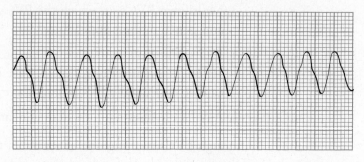

Ventricular tachycardia. The rate is about 200 beats per minute.

The morphology of VT may be uniform, with each complex appearing similar to the one before it, as in the picture above, or it may be polymorphic, changing appearance from beat to beat. Polymorphic VT is more commonly associated with acute coronary ischemia, infarction, profound electrolyte disturbances, and conditions causing prolongation of the QT interval. Uniform VT is more often seen with healed infarctions; the scarred myocardium provides the substrate for the reentrant VT.

Approximately 3.5% of patients develop VT after a myocardial infarction, the large majority within the first 48 hours. An increased risk of VT persists for weeks beyond the myocardial infarction. The development of sustained VT within the first 6 weeks postinfarction is associated with a 1-year mortality rate of about 75%.

Ventricular Fibrillation

Ventricular fibrillation is a preterminal event. It is seen almost solely in dying hearts. It is the most frequently encountered arrhythmia in adults who experience sudden death. The EKG tracing jerks about spasmodically (coarse ventricular fibrillation) or undulates gently (fine ventricular fibrillation). There are no true QRS complexes.

In ventricular fibrillation, the heart generates no cardiac output, and cardiopulmonary resuscitation and electrical defibrillation must be performed at once.

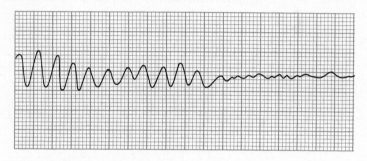

Ventricular tachycardia degenerates into ventricular fibrillation.

Common precipitants of ventricular fibrillation include:

Myocardial ischemia/infarction

Heart failure

Hypoxemia or hypercapnia

Hypotension or shock

Electrolyte imbalances

Stimulants, such as caffeine, alcohol, and drugs

In many cases, ventricular fibrillation is preceded by VT

Accelerated Idioventricular Rhythm

Accelerated idioventricular rhythm is a benign rhythm that is sometimes seen during an acute infarction or during the early hours following reperfusion after an occluded coronary artery has been opened. It is a regular rhythm occurring at 50 to 100 beats per minute and probably represents a ventricular escape focus that has accelerated sufficiently to drive the heart. It is rarely sustained, does not progress to ventricular fibrillation, and rarely requires treatment. When the rate falls below 50 beats per minute, it is then simply called an *idioventricular rhythm* (*i.e.*, the term *accelerated* is dropped).

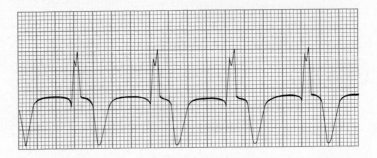

Accelerated idioventricular rhythm. There are no P waves, the QRS complexes are wide, and the rate is about 75 beats per minute.

Torsade de Pointes

Torsade de pointes, meaning "twisting of the points," is more than just the most lyrical name in cardiology. It is a unique form of VT that is usually seen in patients with prolonged QT intervals.

The QT interval, you will recall, encompasses the time from the beginning of ventricular depolarization to the end of ventricular repolarization. It normally constitutes about 40% of the complete cardiac cycle.

A prolonged QT interval can be congenital in origin (resulting from mutations in genes encoding cardiac ion channels), can result from various electrolyte disturbances (notably hypocalcemia, hypomagnesemia, and hypokalemia), or can develop during an acute myocardial infarction. Numerous pharmacologic agents can also prolong the QT interval. These include antiarrhythmic drugs, tricyclic antidepressants, the phenothiazines, and some antifungal medications and antihistamines when taken concurrently with certain antibiotics, particularly erythromycin and the quinolones.

A prolonged QT interval is generally the result of prolonged ventricular repolarization (*i.e.*, the T wave is lengthened). A PVC falling during the elongated T wave can initiate torsade de pointes.

Torsade de pointes looks just like ordinary, run-of-the-mill VT, except that the QRS complexes spiral around the baseline, changing their axis and amplitude. It is important to distinguish torsade de pointes from standard VT because they are treated very differently.

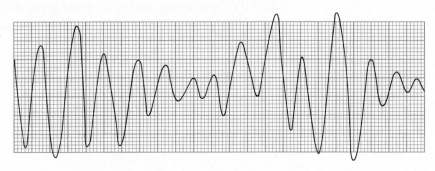

Torsade de pointes. The QRS complexes seem to spin around the baseline, changing their axis and amplitude.

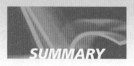

Ventricular Arrhythmias

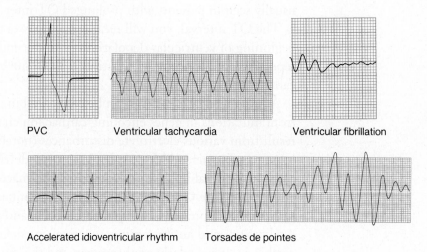

PVC   Ventricular tachycardia   Ventricular fibrillation

Accelerated idioventricular rhythm   Torsades de pointes

Rules of Malignancy for PVCs

Frequent PVCs

Consecutive PVCs

Multiform PVCs

R-on-T phenomenon

Any PVC occurring during an acute myocardial infarction (or in any patient with underlying heart disease)

Supraventricular Versus Ventricular Arrhythmias

The distinction between supraventricular arrhythmias and ventricular arrhythmias is extremely important because the latter generally carry a far more ominous prognosis and the therapy is very different. In most cases, the distinction is simple: supraventricular arrhythmias are associated with a narrow QRS complex, ventricular arrhythmias with a wide QRS complex.

There is one common circumstance, however, in which supraventricular beats can produce wide QRS complexes and make the distinction considerably more difficult. This occurs when a supraventricular beat is conducted aberrantly through the ventricles, producing a wide, bizarre-looking QRS complex that is indistinguishable from a PVC. Here's how it happens.

Aberrancy

Sometimes, an atrial premature beat occurs so early in the next cycle that the Purkinje fibers in the ventricles have not had a chance to repolarize fully in preparation for the next electrical impulse. The right bundle branch, in particular, can be sluggish in this regard, and when the premature atrial impulse reaches the ventricles, the right bundle branch is still refractory. The electrical impulse is therefore prevented from passing down the right bundle branch but is able to pass quite freely down the left bundle branch (figure *A*). Those areas of the ventricular myocardium ordinarily supplied by the right bundle branch must receive their electrical activation from elsewhere, namely from those areas already depolarized by the left bundle branch (figure *B*). The complete process of ventricular depolarization, therefore, takes an unusually long time; the vector of current flow is distorted; and the result is a wide, bizarre QRS complex that looks, for all the world, like a PVC (figure *C*).

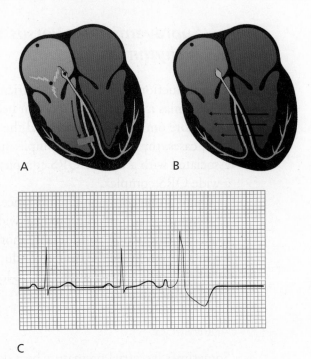

C

(*A*) A premature atrial impulse catches the right bundle branch unprepared. Conduction down the right bundle is blocked but proceeds smoothly down the left bundle. (*B*) Right ventricular depolarization occurs only when the electrical forces can make their way over from the left ventricle—a slow, tedious process. This mode of transmission is very inefficient and results in a wide, bizarre QRS complex. (*C*) The third P wave is a premature atrial contraction. It is conducted aberrantly through the ventricles, generating a wide, bizarre QRS complex.

A wide QRS complex can therefore signify one of two things:

- A beat originating within the ventricles, or

- A supraventricular beat conducted aberrantly

How do you tell the two apart? In the case of a single premature atrial contraction, it's usually easy because there is a P wave preceding the wide QRS complex. Look especially closely at the T wave of the preceding beat to see if a premature P wave is hidden within it. On the other hand, and rather obviously, there is no P wave preceding a PVC.

However, when there are several consecutive beats occurring in rapid succession, or a lengthy, sustained arrhythmia, the distinction can be much more difficult. PSVT and VT have about the same rates. Thus, the tracing below is consistent with either VT or PSVT conducted aberrantly.

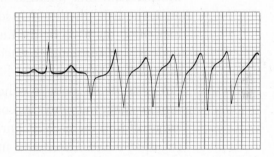

In the tracing above, normal sinus rhythm degenerates into a new rhythm, but is it VT or supraventricular tachycardia conducted aberrantly? Don't feel bad if you can't tell. From this strip alone, as you will see, it is impossible to know for sure.

As you can see from the preceding rhythm strip, it is sometimes impossible to tell these two entities apart. There are, however, several clinical and electrocardiographic clues that can be helpful.

Clinical Clues

1. VT is usually seen in diseased hearts (*e.g.,* in a patient with a prior myocardial infarction or congestive heart failure). PSVT is usually seen in otherwise normal hearts.

2. Carotid massage may terminate PSVT, whereas it has no effect on VT.

3. More than 75% of cases of VT are accompanied by *AV dissociation.* In AV dissociation, the atria and ventricles beat independently of each other. There is a ventricular pacemaker driving the ventricles and producing VT on the EKG, and an independent sinus (or atrial or nodal) pacemaker driving the atria; the atrial rhythm may sometimes be seen but often is not, hidden on the EKG by the much more prominent VT. The AV node is kept constantly refractory by the ceaseless bombardment of impulses from above and below, and therefore no impulse can cross the AV node in either direction. If, as will occur from time to time, the ventricles contract just before the atria, the atria will find themselves contracting against closed mitral and tricuspid valves. This results in a sudden back-flooding of blood into the jugular veins, producing the classic *cannon A waves* of AV dissociation. Cannon A waves are not seen in PSVT.

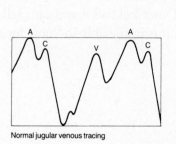 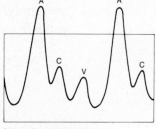

Normal jugular venous tracing

Cannon A waves in a patient with AV dissociation

A wave: right atrial contraction

C wave: closure of the tricuspid valve

V wave: passive filling of the right atrium during diastole

Electrocardiographic Clues

1. AV dissociation accompanying VT can sometimes be seen on the EKG. P waves and QRS complexes march along the rhythm strip completely independently of each other. In PSVT, if P waves are seen, they bear a 1:1 relation to the QRS complexes. And remember, the P waves of PSVT will be retrograde P waves, with a positive deflection in lead AVR and a negative deflection in lead II.

2. *Fusion beats* may be seen in VT only. A fusion beat (or capture beat) occurs when an atrial impulse manages to slip through the AV node at the same time that an impulse of ventricular origin is spreading across the ventricular myocardium. The two impulses jointly depolarize the ventricles, producing a QRS complex that is morphologically part supraventricular and part ventricular.

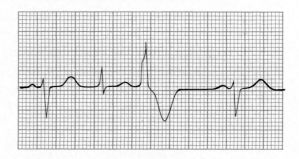

The second beat is a fusion beat, a composite of an atrial (sinus) beat (beats 1 and 4) and a PVC beat (beat 3).

3. In PSVT with aberrancy, the initial deflection of the QRS complex is usually in the same direction as that of the normal QRS complex. In VT, the initial deflection is often in the opposite direction.

None of these criteria is infallible, and sometimes it remains impossible to identify a tachyarrhythmia as ventricular or supraventricular in origin. In patients with recurrent tachycardias whose origin (and, hence, treatment) remains obscure, *electrophysiologic* testing may be necessary (see page 151).

The Ashman Phenomenon

We aren't quite ready to leave the subject of aberrancy. The *Ashman phenomenon* is another example of aberrant conduction of a supraventricular beat. It is commonly seen in patients with atrial fibrillation.

The Ashman phenomenon describes a wide, aberrantly conducted supraventricular beat occurring *after a QRS complex that is preceded by a long pause.*

This is why it happens. The bundle branches reset their rate of repolarization according to the length of the preceding beat. If the preceding beat occurred a relatively long time ago, then the bundles repolarize somewhat leisurely. So imagine a normal beat (the second beat on the tracing below) followed by a long pause before the next beat (the third beat on the tracing). The bundle branches anticipate another long pause following this beat and repolarize slowly. If, before repolarization is complete, another supraventricular impulse should pass through the AV node, conduction will be blocked along one of the normal bundle branch pathways, and a wide, bizarre QRS complex will be inscribed (the fourth and obviously abnormal beat).

Atrial fibrillation, with its variable conduction producing long and short pauses between QRS complexes, is the perfect setting for this to occur.

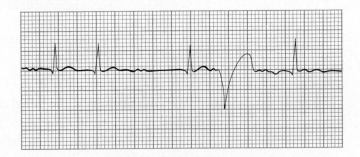

The Ashman phenomenon. The fourth beat looks like a PVC, but it could also be an aberrantly conducted supraventricular beat. Note the underlying atrial fibrillation, the short interval before the second beat, and the long interval before the third beat—all in all, a perfect substrate for the Ashman phenomenon.

Fortunately, most supraventricular arrhythmias are associated with narrow QRS complexes; aberrancy, although not uncommon, is at least the exception, not the rule. The point to take home is this: a narrow QRS complex virtually always implies a supraventricular origin, whereas a wide QRS complex usually implies a ventricular origin but may reflect aberrant conduction of a supraventricular beat.

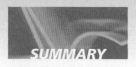

Ventricular Tachycardia (VT) Versus PSVT With Aberrancy

	VT	*PSVT*
Clinical Clues		
Clinical history	Diseased heart	Usually healthy heart
Carotid massage	No response	May terminate
Cannon A waves	May be present	Not seen
EKG Clues		
AV dissociation	May be seen	Not seen
Fusion beats	May be seen	Not seen
Initial QRS deflection	May differ from normal QRS complex	Same as normal QRS complex

Programmed Electrical Stimulation

Programmed electrical stimulation (abbreviated EPS for electrophysiologic studies) has added a new dimension to the treatment of arrhythmias. Before the introduction of EPS, a patient with an arrhythmia requiring treatment was given a drug empirically, and after several days, when therapeutic levels had been achieved, a 24-hour Holter monitor would be used to see whether the frequency of the arrhythmia had been reduced. This hit-or-miss approach was time-consuming and exposed patients to the potential side effects of drugs that might prove of no benefit.

EPS is certainly not necessary for all patients with arrhythmias, and the Holter monitor remains the staple of arrhythmia diagnosis and treatment. EPS is expensive and invasive, but for certain patients it has great value, greatly refining the process of choosing the right drug for patients who need rapid and effective therapy.

The patient is taken to the electrophysiology laboratory where the particular arrhythmia is induced with intracardiac electrodes. Tiny catheters are inserted through peripheral veins or arteries and are then advanced to various locations within the chambers of the heart. A catheter placed at the junction of the right atrium and ventricle at the upper posterior portion of the tricuspid ring will record a His bundle potential, which can help to define the electrical relationship of the atria and ventricles during the propagation of an arrhythmia. For example, if with atrial activation a His potential precedes every QRS complex, then a supraventricular origin is likely. In this way, the source of an arrhythmia can be mapped to determine the most appropriate therapy.

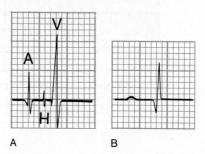

(*A*) A His bundle recording and (*B*) the corresponding EKG. In *A*, the small spike (H) between the spikes of atrial (A) and ventricular (V) activation reflects activation of the bundle of His.

EPS has been used most successfully in patients who have recurrent VT or who have experienced a previous episode of sudden death requiring cardiopulmonary resuscitation.

EPS mapping techniques have become extremely precise, and the technique of *catheter ablation* often mitigates the need for a more extensive surgical procedure. With this technique, it is possible to intentionally damage (*ablate*) a portion of the reentrant pathway that is the origin of the rhythm disturbance by applying electrical energy (most commonly radiofrequency) to where the catheter tip is in contact with the myocardium. Catheter ablation usually results in a permanent cure, leaving only a 4- or 5-mm scar, and the patient may not even require medication.

Implantable Defibrillators

Even when EPS-guided drug therapies or catheter ablation techniques are used, the recurrence rates for VT are still unacceptably high. For this reason, *implantable cardioverter–defibrillators* have become the standard form of protection for most patients with life-threatening arrhythmias. These small devices are surgically implanted, like a pacemaker, under the skin below the clavicle. There they continuously monitor the heart rhythm and, when they sense a dangerous arrhythmia, deliver an electric shock to the heart through an electrode that rests in the right ventricle.

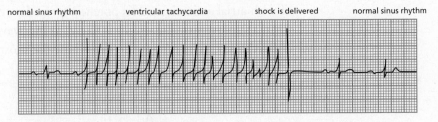

normal sinus rhythm   ventricular tachycardia   shock is delivered   normal sinus rhythm

The heart rate of a 72-year-old woman is rescued from VT by a shock delivered by an implantable cardioverter–defibrillator.

External Defibrillators

Automatic external defibrillators are small portable devices that come equipped with patches that attach to the chest wall. Once hooked up, these devices can quickly determine whether the rhythm of an individual who has collapsed is ventricular fibrillation and, if so, can deliver defibrillation shocks that may be lifesaving. Minimal training is required to learn how to operate the defibrillator and place the patches properly. They are now widely available in police cars, on airplanes, and in public venues.

Here is an opportunity to review the arrhythmias we have been discussing. If you want to reexamine the basic characteristics of each arrhythmia before trying these examples, go back to the sections on arrhythmias of sinus origin, supraventricular arrhythmias, and ventricular arrhythmias. For each tracing, use the four-step method discussed previously. Always ask the following questions:

1. Are P waves present?

2. Are the QRS complexes narrow or wide?

3. What is the relationship between the P waves and QRS complexes?

4. Is the rhythm regular or irregular?

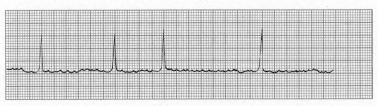

A

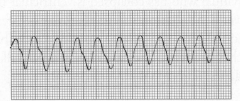

B

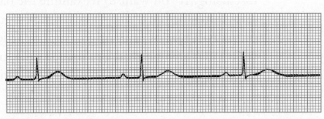

C

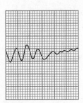

D

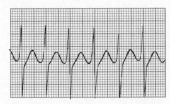

E

(A) Atrial fibrillation. (B) Ventricular tachycardia. (C) Sinus bradycardia. (D) VT degenerating into ventricular fibrillation. (E) PSVT.

CASE

3.

Lola deB., predictably, is the life of the party. Never missing a turn on the dance floor nor a round at the bar, she becomes increasingly intoxicated as the evening progresses. Her husband, a young business executive, forces her to drink some coffee to sober her up before they leave. As he is wandering around in search of their coats, he hears a scream and rushes back to find her collapsed on the floor. Everyone is in a panic and all eyes turn to you, word having gotten around that you have recently been reading a well-known and highly regarded EKG book. The terror in the room is palpable, but you grin modestly, toss down a final swig of mineral water, and stride confidently to the patient saying as you go, "Don't worry. I can handle it."

Can you? What has happened to Lola, and just what are you going to do about it?

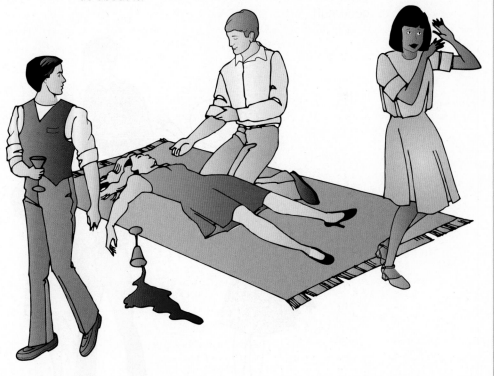

Of course, a whole host of things could have happened to Lola (they usually do), but you know that the combination of alcohol, coffee, and the excitement of the party can induce a PSVT in anyone, no matter how healthy they are and no matter how normal their heart. It is likely that this supraventricular rhythm disturbance has caused her to faint.

You bend down over her, assure yourself that she is breathing, and feel her pulse. It is rapid and regular with a rate of about 200 beats per minute. Because she is young and very unlikely to have significant carotid artery disease, you go right ahead and perform carotid massage, and within about 10 seconds you feel her pulse shift gears and return to normal. Her eyes blink open and the room erupts in cheers. Your guess was correct.

As you are carried out of the room on everyone's shoulders, don't forget to remind them which book you were reading that taught you all this good stuff.

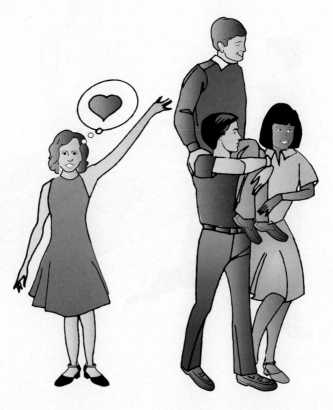

In patients with tachyarrhythmias that result in syncope, further evaluation is usually warranted because of the high likelihood of recurrence. This evaluation usually includes at least appropriate laboratory studies (*e.g.*, to rule out electrolyte imbalances and hyperthyroidism), a stress-cardiac echo (to look for valvular disease and coronary artery disease; see page 254 on stress testing), and a Holter monitor or event recorder to capture any further rhythm disturbances. Seizure activity associated with the syncopal event or any persistent neurologic deficits will necessitate a full neurologic evaluation. In many states and countries, if no treatable cause for the syncopal event is found, the patient will not be permitted to drive for at least several months.

CASE

4.

George M., irascible and older than time, comes to see you late one Friday afternoon (he always comes late on Friday afternoons, probably because he knows you like to get an early start on the weekend). This time he tells you that he fainted the day before and now is feeling a bit light-headed. He also has a strange fluttering sensation in his chest. George is always complaining of something, and you have yet to find anything the matter with him in the many years you have known him, but just to be careful you obtain an EKG.

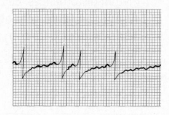

You quickly recognize the arrhythmia and are reaching for your stethoscope when George's eyes roll back in his head and he drops unconscious to the floor. Fortunately, the EKG is still running, and you see

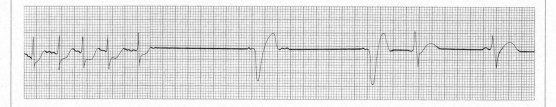

You drop down to his side, ready, if need be, to begin cardiopulmonary resuscitation, when his eyes pop open and he mutters something under his breath. The EKG now shows

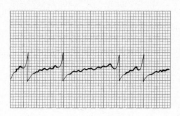

You may not know what's going on, but at least you can identify the three tracings. Right?

The first and third tracings are the same, showing classic atrial fibrillation. The baseline is undulating, without clear-cut P waves, and the QRS complexes appear irregularly. The second tracing is more interesting. It shows the atrial fibrillation terminating abruptly and then a long pause. (It was during such a pause that George dropped to the floor, a result of brain hypoxia caused by the lack of significant cardiac output.) The beats that you see next are ventricular escape beats. The QRS complexes are wide and bizarre, there are no P waves, and the rate is about 33 beats per minute, exactly what you would expect of a ventricular escape rhythm. The final thing you see on the strip is the sinus node at last kicking in, albeit at a slow rate of 50 beats per minute.

George has sick sinus syndrome, also called the bradytachycardia syndrome. It is typified by alternating episodes of a supraventricular tachycardia, such as atrial fibrillation, and bradycardia. Often, when the supraventricular arrhythmia terminates, there is a long pause (greater than 4 seconds) before the sinus node fires again (hence, the term sick sinus). Fortunately for George, a few ventricular escape beats came to a timely rescue. Sick sinus syndrome usually reflects significant underlying disease of the conduction system of the sort that we are studying in the next chapter. It is one of the leading reasons for pacemaker insertion.

George M. revives in your office and insists on going home. Fortunately, wiser heads prevail and he is taken by ambulance to the hospital. A short stay in the CCU confirms that he has not had a heart attack, but his heart monitor shows numerous episodes of prolonged bradycardia alternating with various supraventricular arrhythmias. It is decided that George should have a pacemaker placed, and he reluctantly agrees. The pacemaker provides a safety net, giving George's heart an electrical "kick" every time his own electrical mechanism fails him. George is discharged, and no further episodes of symptomatic bradycardia occur.

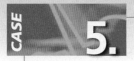

CASE 5. Frederick vanZ is a renowned (and highly strung) orchestral conductor whose delusions of grandeur are tempered by a small regular dose of halo-peridol, a commonly prescribed antipsychotic medication. Late one night, after an all-Beethoven performance at the large concert hall in your town, he is rushed to the hospital with a high fever, confusion, and blood in his urine (hematuria). In the emergency room, he is found to be hypotensive from urosepsis. He is immediately treated with the intravenous antibiotic, levofloxacin. Here is lead II from his cardiac monitor in the emergency room. Can you identify his rhythm?

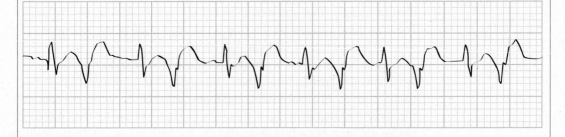

You should recognize two different types of beats of very different morphology, alternating with one another. The maestro is in bigeminy, with supraventricular beats (junctional beats, with a narrow QRS complex and no visible P wave) occurring in a 1:1 ratio with ventricular beats (PVCs, with a wide QRS complex).

He is transferred to the intensive care unit where you confidently take over his case. As soon as you hook him up to the heart monitor, you see this. What has happened?

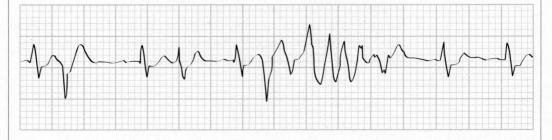

Let's read this left to right. The first beat is a junctional beat, the second a PVC, and the third and fourth beats two more junctional beats. He clearly is no longer in strict bigeminy. On the fifth beat, right after the QRS complex, a PVC has landed on the vulnerable QT interval and triggered a short run of a VT that is fortunately self-terminating.

Moments later, his blood pressure collapses, his body seizes up in bed, and you see the following arrhythmia. In a flash, you recognize it and prepare to swing into action. What does the tracing show?

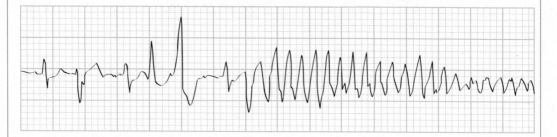

As in the previous tracing, a PVC has fallen on a QT interval, but now the resulting VT persists. The changes in amplitude (reflecting a change in axis as the QRS complexes spiral around the baseline) identify the arrhythmia as torsade de pointes, a medical emergency.

The great conductor is successfully treated (urgent temporary cardiac pacing does the trick), and his vital signs return to normal. Several hours later, his rhythm strip now shows this. Please identify the rhythm and look closely at the lengths of the various intervals:

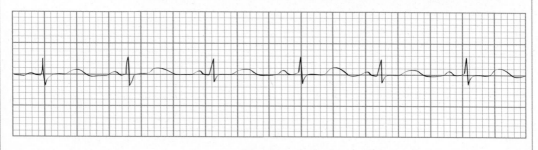

He is in normal sinus rhythm—note the first appearance of P waves—but take a close look at his QT interval. Normally, it should comprise about 40% of the cardiac cycle, but here it measures well over 50% of one cardiac cycle. This prolonged QT interval was the perfect substrate for torsade de pointes. The patient was on two drugs that can prolong the QT interval—haloperidol, which he was taking on a chronic basis, and levofloxacin, the antibiotic he was given in the emergency room that acutely lengthened his QT interval even more and set up the great master for the nearly fatal events that followed. You immediately discontinue both medications, and his QT interval normalizes. There will be no more episodes of torsade de pointes on your watch!

4. Conduction Blocks

In this chapter you will learn:

1 | what a conduction block is

2 | that there are several types of conduction blocks that can occur between the sinus node and the atrioventricular (AV) node, some that are of little concern and others that can be life threatening

3 | how to recognize each of these AV blocks on the EKG

4 | that conduction blocks can occur in the ventricles as well, and these bundle branch blocks are also easily identified on the EKG

5 | that sometimes conduction along only one fascicle of a bundle branch can be blocked

6 | how to recognize combined AV blocks and bundle branch blocks on the EKG

7 | what pacemakers are used for, and how to recognize their bursts of electrical activity on an EKG

8 | about the case of Sally M., which will illustrate the importance of knowing when conduction disturbances are truly disturbing.

What Is a Conduction Block?

Any obstruction or delay of the flow of electricity along the normal pathways of electrical conduction is called a *conduction block*.

A conduction block can occur anywhere in the conduction system of the heart. There are three types of conduction blocks, defined by their anatomic location.

1. *Sinus node block*—This is the sinus exit block that we discussed in the last chapter. In this situation, the sinus node fires normally, but the wave of depolarization is immediately blocked and is not transmitted into the atrial tissue. On the EKG, it looks just like a pause in the normal cardiac cycle. We will not discuss it further.

2. *Atrioventricular (AV) block*—This term refers to any conduction block between the sinus node and the Purkinje fibers. Note that this includes the AV node and His bundle.

3. *Bundle branch block*—As the name indicates, bundle branch block refers to a conduction block in one or both of the ventricular bundle branches. Sometimes, only a part of one of the bundle branches is blocked; this circumstance is called a *fascicular block* or a *hemiblock*.

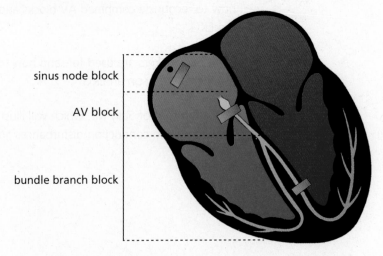

sinus node block

AV block

bundle branch block

To a rough approximation, this picture shows typical sites of the three major conduction blocks.

AV Blocks

AV blocks come in three varieties, termed (with a complete lack of imagination) *first degree, second degree,* and *third degree.* They are diagnosed by carefully examining the relationship of the P waves to the QRS complexes.

First-Degree AV Block

First-degree AV block is characterized by a prolonged delay in conduction at the AV node or His bundle (recall that the His bundle— or bundle of His, depending on your grammatical preference—is the part of the conducting system located just below the AV node. A routine 12-lead EKG cannot distinguish between a block in the AV node and one in the His bundle). The wave of depolarization spreads normally from the sinus node through the atria, but upon reaching the AV node is held up for longer than the usual one-tenth of a second. As a result, the PR interval—the time between the start of atrial depolarization and the start of ventricular depolarization, the time period that encompasses the delay at the AV node—is prolonged.

The diagnosis of first-degree AV block requires only that the PR interval be longer than 0.2 seconds.

In first-degree AV block, despite the delay at the AV node or His bundle, every atrial impulse does eventually make it through the AV node to activate the ventricles. Therefore, to be precise, first-degree AV block is not really a "block" at all, but rather a "delay" in conduction. Every QRS complex is preceded by a single P wave.

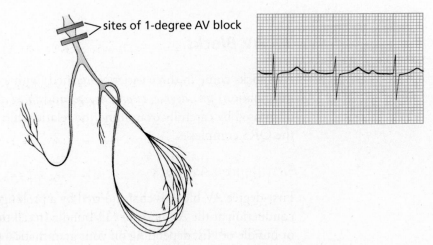

First-degree AV block. Note the prolonged PR interval.

First-degree AV block is a common finding in normal hearts, but it can also be an early sign of degenerative disease of the conduction system or a transient manifestation of myocarditis or drug toxicity. By itself, it does not require treatment. However, first-degree AV block is associated with an increased risk of atrial fibrillation, the need for subsequent pacemaker insertion, and all-cause mortality. The reason for this is not clear but may reflect the possibility that a prolonged PR interval is a precursor to more severe heart block or is a marker for underlying cardiovascular disease.

Second-Degree AV Block

In *second-degree AV block,* not every atrial impulse is able to pass through the AV node into the ventricles. Because some P waves fail to conduct through to the ventricles, the ratio of P waves to QRS complexes is greater than 1:1.

Just to make things a little more interesting, there are two types of second-degree AV block: *Mobitz type I second-degree AV block,* more commonly called *Wenckebach block,* and *Mobitz type II second-degree AV block.*

Wenckebach Block

Wenckebach block is almost always due to a block *within* the AV node. However, the electrical effects of Wenckebach block are unique. The block, or delay, is variable, increasing with each ensuing impulse. **Each successive atrial impulse encounters a longer and longer delay in the AV node until one impulse (usually every third or fourth) fails to make it through.** What you see on the EKG is a progressive lengthening of the PR interval with each beat and then suddenly a P wave that is not followed by a QRS complex (a "dropped beat"). After this dropped beat, during which no QRS complex appears, the sequence repeats itself, over and over, and often with impressive regularity.

The following tracing shows a 4:3 Wenckebach block, in which the PR interval grows longer with each beat until the fourth atrial impulse fails to stimulate the ventricles, producing a ratio of four P waves to every three QRS complexes.

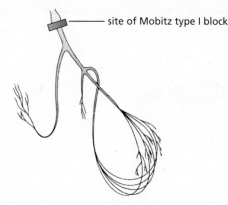

site of Mobitz type I block

Mobitz type I second-degree AV block (Wenckebach block). The PR intervals become progressively longer until one QRS complex is dropped.

The diagnosis of Wenckebach block requires the progressive lengthening of each successive PR interval until one P wave fails to conduct through the AV node and is therefore not followed by a QRS complex.

Mobitz Type II Block

Mobitz type II block is usually due to a block *below* the AV node in the His bundle. It resembles Wenckebach block in that some, but not all, of the atrial impulses are transmitted to the ventricles. However, progressive lengthening of the PR interval does not occur. Instead, conduction is an all-or-nothing phenomenon. The EKG shows two or more normal beats with normal PR intervals and then a P wave that is not followed by a QRS complex (a dropped beat). The cycle is then repeated. The ratio of conducted beats to nonconducted beats is rarely constant, with the ratio of P waves to QRS complexes constantly varying, from 2:1 to 3:2 and so on.

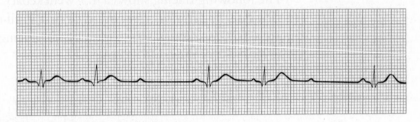

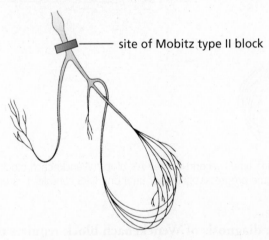

site of Mobitz type II block

Mobitz type II second-degree AV block. On this EKG, each third P wave is not followed by a QRS complex (dropped beat).

The diagnosis of Mobitz type II block requires the presence of a dropped beat without progressive lengthening of the PR interval.

Is It a Wenckebach Block or a Mobitz Type II Block?

Compare the electrocardiographic manifestations of Wenckebach block and Mobitz type II block on the following EKGs:

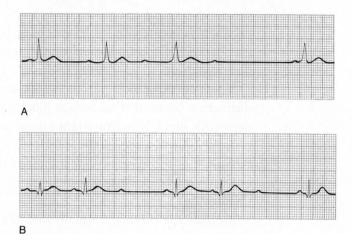

A

B

(*A*) Wenckebach block, with progressive lengthening of the PR interval.
(*B*) Mobitz type II block, in which the PR interval is constant.

Now that you are an expert, look at the following EKG. Is this an example of Wenckebach block or Mobitz type II block?

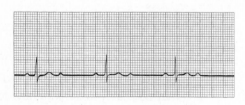

Well, it certainly is an example of second-degree heart block with a P wave–to–QRS complex ratio of 2:1, but you were pretty clever if you realized that it is impossible to tell whether it is due to Wenckebach block or Mobitz type II block. The distinction between these two types of second-degree heart block depends on whether or not there is progressive PR lengthening; but with a 2:1 ratio in which every other QRS complex is dropped, it is impossible to make this determination.

When circumstances permit a more accurate determination, the distinction between Wenckebach block and Mobitz type II second-degree AV block is an important one to make. Wenckebach block is usually due to a conduction block high up in the AV node. It is typically transient and benign and rarely progresses to third-degree heart block (see next page), which can be dangerous and even life threatening.

Mobitz type II block is usually due to a conduction block below the AV node, somewhere in the His bundle. Although less common than Wenckebach block, it is far more serious, often signifying serious heart disease and capable of progressing suddenly to third-degree heart block.

Whereas treatment is often not needed for Wenckebach block, Mobitz type II heart block often mandates insertion of a pacemaker.

Here is a little technical esoterica that, unless you plan to become a cardiologist, you can probably safely ignore. In cases of 2:1 second-degree AV block, as shown on the previous page, there is a way to localize the site of the block and determine how serious the problem may be. Can you think of how to do it?

His bundle electrocardiography, as described previously, will do the job. A small electrode introduced into the region of the His bundle can identify whether the site of the block is above, within, or below the His bundle and therefore can accurately predict the patient's prognosis; that is, the likelihood of progression to third-degree heart block.

Third-Degree AV Block

Third-degree heart block is the ultimate in heart blocks. No atrial impulses make it through to activate the ventricles. For this reason, it is often called *complete heart block*. The site of the block can be either at the AV node or lower. The ventricles respond to this dire situation by generating an escape rhythm, usually an inadequate 30 to 45 beats per minute (idioventricular escape). The atria and ventricles continue to contract, but they now do so at their own intrinsic rates—about 60 to 100 beats per minute for the atria and 30 to 45 beats per minute for the ventricles. In complete heart block, the atria and ventricles have virtually nothing to do with each other, separated by the absolute barrier of the complete conduction block. We have already described this type of situation in our discussion of ventricular tachycardia: it is called *AV dissociation* and refers to any circumstance in which the atria and ventricles are being driven by independent pacemakers.

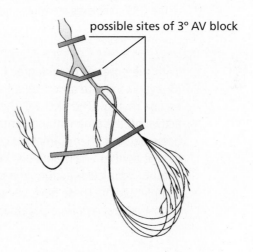

possible sites of 3° AV block

The EKG in third-degree heart block shows P waves marching across the rhythm strip at their usual rate (60 to 100 waves per minute) but bearing no relationship to the QRS complexes that appear at a much slower escape rate. The QRS complexes appear wide and bizarre, just like premature ventricular contraction (PVCs), because they arise from a ventricular source.

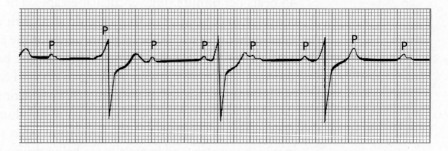

Third-degree AV block. The P waves appear at regular intervals, as do the QRS complexes, but they have nothing to do with one another. The QRS complexes are wide, implying a ventricular origin.

With the onset of third-degree heart block, there may be a delay (or even complete absence) in the appearance of a ventricular escape rhythm. The EKG will then show sinus beats (P waves) activating the atria with no ventricular activity at all for two or more beats before either normal AV conduction resumes or a ventricular escape rhythm finally appears. When there are 4 or more seconds without ventricular activity, the patient usually experiences a near or complete faint. These have been termed Stokes-Adams attacks and almost always require a pacemaker (see page 195).

Although a ventricular escape rhythm may look like a slow run of PVCs (slow ventricular tachycardia), there is one important difference: PVCs are *premature,* occurring before the next expected beat, and even the slowest VT will be faster than the patient's normal rhythm. A ventricular escape beat occurs after a long pause and is therefore never premature, and a sustained ventricular escape rhythm is always *slower* than the normal beats. PVCs, being premature intrusions, can be suppressed with little clinical consequence. A ventricular escape rhythm, however, may be lifesaving, and suppression could be fatal.

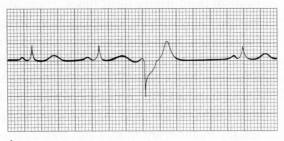

A

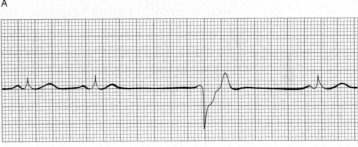

B

(*A*) The third beat is a PVC, occurring before the next anticipated normal beat. (*B*) The third ventricular complex occurs late, after a prolonged pause. This is a ventricular escape beat.

The diagnosis of third-degree heart block requires the presence of AV dissociation in which the ventricular rate is slower than the sinus or atrial rate.

AV dissociation can also occur when there is a block high in the AV node, but in this case, there is an accelerated junctional rhythm to drive the ventricles that is faster than the sinus rhythm. This situation rarely requires a pacemaker. It occurs most often in patients undergoing an acute infarction and those who have received an overdose of an antiarrhythmic medication.

Degenerative disease of the conduction system is the leading cause of third-degree heart block. It can also complicate an acute myocardial infarction. Pacemakers are virtually always required when third-degree heart block develops. It is a true medical emergency.

A common cause of *reversible* complete heart block is Lyme disease. The heart block typically occurs within the AV node and is associated with a narrow QRS complex *junctional* escape rhythm. A stat Lyme titer can avoid the need for a permanent pacemaker. Treatment usually includes antibiotics and corticosteroids.

Some forms of complete heart block develop prenatally (congenital heart block), and these are often associated with an adequate and stable ventricular escape rhythm. Permanent pacemakers are only implanted in these children if there is clear-cut developmental impairment that can be attributed to an inadequate cardiac output.

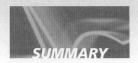

AV Blocks

AV block is diagnosed by examining the relationship of the P waves to the QRS complexes.

1. *First degree:* The PR interval is greater than 0.2 seconds; *all* beats are conducted through to the ventricles.

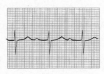

2. *Second degree:* Only *some* beats are conducted through to the ventricles.

   a. *Mobitz type I* (Wenckebach): Progressive prolongation of the PR interval until a QRS is dropped

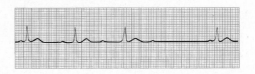

   b. *Mobitz type II:* All-or-nothing conduction, in which QRS complexes are dropped without prolongation of the PR interval

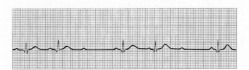

3. *Third degree:* No beats are conducted through to the ventricles. There is complete heart block with AV dissociation, in which the atria and ventricles are driven by independent pacemakers.

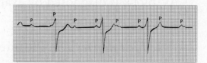

Note: Different degrees of AV block can coexist in the same patient. Thus, for example, a patient can have both first-degree and Mobitz type II heart block. Blocks also can be transient—a patient may, for example, at one point have a second-degree block that later progresses to third-degree block.

Bundle Branch Block

The term *bundle branch block* refers to a conduction block in either the left or right bundle branches. The following figure reviews the anatomy of the ventricular bundle branches.

A Quick Review of Ventricular Depolarization

The normal sequence of ventricular activation should be familiar to you by now. The wave of depolarization sweeps out of the AV node and bundle of His into the bundle branch system. The right and left bundle branches deliver the current to the right and left ventricles, respectively. This is the most efficient means of dispersing the electrical current, and the resultant QRS complex, representing ventricular depolarization from start to finish, is narrow—less than 0.10 seconds in duration. Also, because the muscle mass of the left ventricle is so much larger than that of the right ventricle, left ventricular electrical forces dominate those of the right ventricle, and the resultant electrical axis is leftward, lying between 0° and +90°.

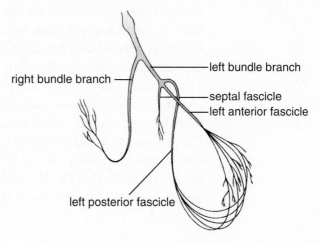

The anatomy of the ventricular bundle branches.

Thus, with normal ventricular depolarization, the QRS complex is narrow, and the electrical axis lies between 0° and 90°. *All of this changes with bundle branch block.*

Bundle branch block is diagnosed by looking at the width and configuration of the QRS complexes.

Right Bundle Branch Block

In *right bundle branch block,* conduction through the right bundle is obstructed. As a result, right ventricular depolarization is delayed; it does not begin until the left ventricle is almost fully depolarized. This causes two things to happen on the EKG:

1. The delay in right ventricular depolarization prolongs the total time for ventricular depolarization. As a result, the QRS complex widens beyond 0.12 seconds.

2. The wide QRS complex assumes a unique, virtually diagnostic shape in those leads overlying the right ventricle: V1 and V2. The *normal* QRS complex in these leads consists of a small positive R wave and a deep negative S wave, reflecting the electrical dominance of the left ventricle. With *right bundle branch block*, you can still see the initial R and S waves as the left ventricle depolarizes, but as the right ventricle then begins its delayed depolarization, unopposed by the now fully depolarized and electrically silent left ventricle, the electrical axis of current flow swings sharply back toward the right. This inscribes a *second* R wave, called R′ (pronounced "R prime"), in leads V1 and V2. The whole complex is called RSR′ ("R-S-R prime"), and its appearance has been likened to rabbit ears. Meanwhile, in the left lateral leads overlying the left ventricle (I, aVL, V5, and V6), late right ventricular depolarization causes reciprocal late deep S waves to be inscribed.

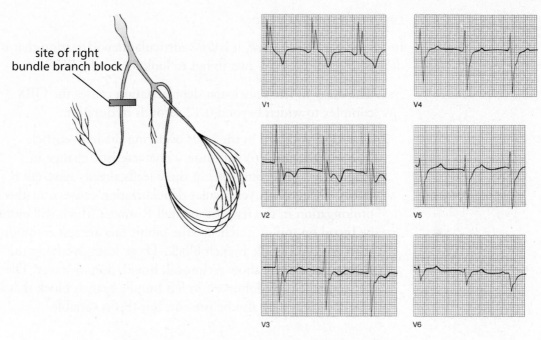

site of right
bundle branch block

Right bundle branch block. The QRS complex in lead V1 shows the 'classic wide RSR' configuration. Note, too, the S waves in V5 and V6.

Left Bundle Branch Block

In *left bundle branch block,* it is *left* ventricular depolarization that is delayed. Again, there are two things to look for on the EKG:

1. The delay in left ventricular depolarization causes the QRS complex to widen beyond 0.12 seconds in duration.

2. The QRS complex in the leads overlying the left ventricle (I, aVL, V5, and V6) will show a characteristic change in shape. The QRS complexes in these leads already have tall R waves. Delayed left ventricular depolarization causes a marked prolongation in the rise of those tall R waves, which will either be broad on top or notched. True rabbit ears are less common than in right bundle branch block. Those leads overlying the right ventricle will show reciprocal, broad, deep S waves. The left ventricle is so dominant in left bundle branch block that left axis deviation may also be present, but this is variable.

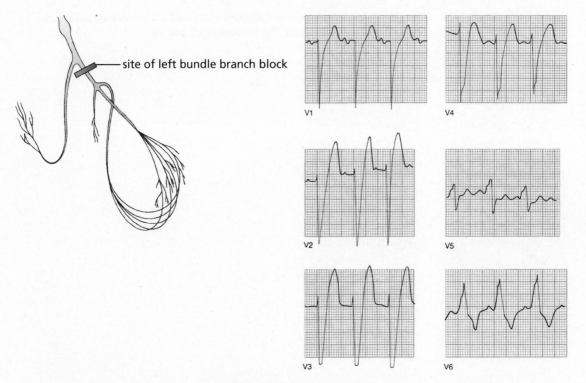

site of left bundle branch block

Left bundle branch block.

Bundle Branch Block and Repolarization

In both right and left bundle branch block, the repolarization sequence is also affected.

In right bundle branch block, the right precordial leads will show ST segment depression and T wave inversion, just like the repolarization abnormalities that occur with ventricular hypertrophy.

Similarly, in left bundle branch block, ST segment depression and T wave inversion can be seen in the left lateral leads.

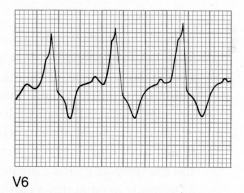

V6

ST segment depression and T wave inversion in lead V6 in a patient with left bundle branch block.

Who Gets Bundle Branch Blocks?

Although right bundle branch block can be caused by diseases of the conducting system, it is also a fairly common phenomenon in otherwise normal hearts.

Left bundle branch block, on the other hand, rarely occurs in normal hearts and almost always reflects significant underlying cardiac disease, such as degenerative disease of the conduction system or ischemic coronary artery disease.

Critical Rate

Both right and left bundle branch block can be intermittent or fixed. In some individuals, bundle branch block only appears when a particular heart rate, called the *critical rate*, is achieved. In other words, the ventricles conduct normally at slow heart rates, but above a certain rate, bundle branch block develops.

The development of a rate-related bundle branch block is directly related to the time it takes a particular bundle branch to repolarize and thus prepare itself for the next electrical impulse to arrive. If the heart rate is so rapid that a particular bundle branch cannot repolarize in time, there will be a temporary block to conduction, resulting in the classic EKG appearance of a rate-related bundle branch block.

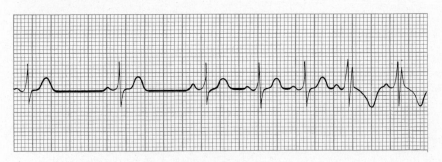

An example of critical rate (lead V2). As the heart accelerates, the pattern of right bundle branch block appears.

The occurrence of rate-related bundle branch block depends on the same physiology that accounts for aberrant conduction of supraventricular arrhythmias (see page 148), in which the aberrantly conducted supraventricular beat results from some portion of the bundle branch system failing to repolarize in a timely fashion.

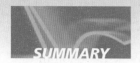

SUMMARY

Bundle Branch Block

Bundle branch block is diagnosed by looking at the width and configuration of the QRS complexes.

Criteria for Right Bundle Branch Block

1. QRS complex widened to greater than 0.12 seconds

2. RSR' in V1 and V2 (rabbit ears) with ST segment depression and T wave inversion

3. Reciprocal changes in V5, V6, I, and aVL.

Criteria for Left Bundle Branch Block

1. QRS complex widened to greater than 0.12 seconds

2. Broad or notched R wave with prolonged upstroke in leads V5, V6, I, and aVL, with ST segment depression and T wave inversion

3. Reciprocal changes in V1 and V2

4. Left axis deviation may be present.

Note: Because bundle branch block affects the size and appearance of R waves, the criteria for ventricular hypertrophy discussed in Chapter 2 cannot be used if bundle branch block is present. Specifically, right bundle branch block precludes the diagnosis of right ventricular hypertrophy, and left bundle branch block precludes the diagnosis of left ventricular hypertrophy. In addition, the diagnosis of a myocardial infarction can be extremely difficult in the presence of left bundle branch block; we will see why in Chapter 6.

Hemiblocks

Here again is a picture of the ventricular conduction system. The left bundle branch is composed of three separate fascicles—the septal fascicle, the left anterior fascicle, and the left posterior fascicle. The term *hemiblock* refers to a conduction block of just one of these fascicles. The right bundle branch does not divide into separate fascicles; thus, the concept of hemiblock only applies to the left ventricular conducting system.

Septal blocks need not concern us here. Hemiblocks of the anterior and posterior fascicles, however, are both common and important.

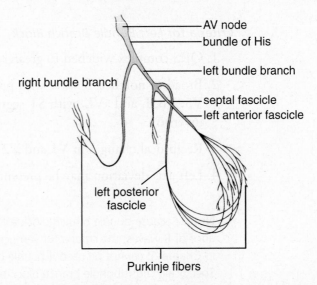

The ventricular conduction system. The right bundle branch remains intact, whereas the left bundle branch divides into three separate fascicles.

Hemiblocks Cause Axis Deviation

The major effect that hemiblocks have on the EKG is *axis deviation*. Here is why.

As shown on the previous page, the left anterior fascicle lies superiorly and laterally to the left posterior fascicle. With *left anterior hemiblock,* conduction down the left anterior fascicle is blocked. All the current, therefore, rushes down the left posterior fascicle to the inferior surface of the heart. Left ventricular myocardial depolarization then occurs, progressing in an inferior-to-superior and right-to-left direction.

The axis of ventricular depolarization is therefore redirected upward and slightly leftward, inscribing tall positive R waves in the left lateral leads and deep S waves inferiorly. This results in *left axis deviation* in which the electrical axis of ventricular depolarization is redirected between –30° and +90°.

Do you remember how to identify left axis deviation? The simplest method is to look at the QRS complex in leads I and aVF. The QRS complex will be positive in lead I and negative in lead aVF. However, this analysis will define a range from 0° to –90°. Therefore, look at lead II, which is angled at +60°; if its QRS complex is negative, then the axis must lie more negative than –30°.

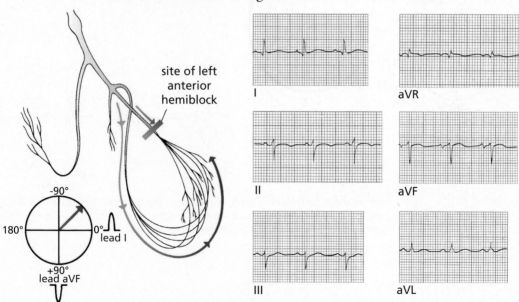

Left anterior hemiblock. Current flow down the left anterior fascicle is blocked; hence, all the current must pass down the posterior fascicle. The resultant axis is redirected upward and leftward (left axis deviation).

In *left posterior hemiblock,* the reverse occurs. All of the current rushes down the left anterior fascicle, and ventricular myocardial depolarization then ensues in a superior-to-inferior and left-to-right direction. The axis of depolarization is therefore directed downward and rightward, writing tall R waves inferiorly and deep S waves in the left lateral leads. The result is *right axis deviation (i.e.,* the electrical axis of ventricular depolarization is between +90° and 180°). The QRS complex will be negative in lead I and positive in lead aVF.

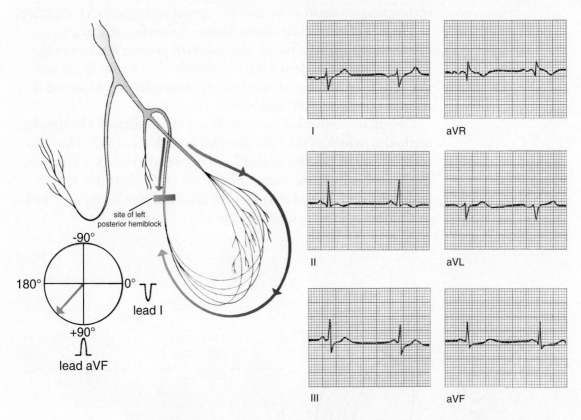

Left posterior hemiblock. Current flow down the left posterior fascicle is blocked; hence, all the current must pass down the right anterior fascicle. The resultant axis is redirected downward and rightward (right axis deviation).

Hemiblocks Do Not Prolong the QRS Complex

Whereas the QRS complex is widened in *complete* left and right bundle branch block, the QRS duration in both left anterior and left posterior hemiblock is normal. (Actually, there is a very minor prolongation, but not enough to widen the QRS complex appreciably.) There are also no ST segment and T wave changes.

Left anterior hemiblock is far more common than left posterior hemiblock, possibly because the anterior fascicle is longer and thinner and has a more tenuous blood supply than the posterior fascicle. Left anterior hemiblock can be seen in both normal and diseased hearts, whereas left posterior hemiblock is virtually the exclusive province of sick hearts.

Is hemiblock present in the following EKG?

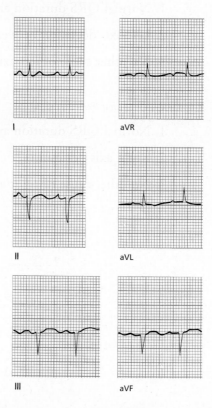

Left axis deviation greater than −30° indicates the presence of left anterior hemiblock.

Before settling on the diagnosis of hemiblock, it is always necessary to make sure that other causes of axis deviation, such as ventricular hypertrophy, are not present. In addition, as we shall discuss later, patients with certain clinical disorders, such as those with severe chronic lung disease, can develop right axis deviation. Nevertheless, for most individuals, if the tracing is normal except for the presence of axis deviation, you can feel reasonably confident that hemiblock is responsible.

Criteria for Hemiblock

Hemiblock is diagnosed by looking for left or right axis deviation.

Left Anterior Hemiblock

1. Normal QRS duration and no ST segment or T wave changes

2. Left axis deviation between –30° and +90°

3. No other cause of left axis deviation is present.

Left Posterior Hemiblock

1. Normal QRS duration and no ST segment or T wave changes

2. Right axis deviation

3. No other cause of right axis deviation is present.

Combining Right Bundle Branch Block and Hemiblocks

Right bundle branch block and hemiblocks can occur together. The term *bifascicular block* refers to the combination of either left anterior or left posterior hemiblock with right bundle branch block. In bifascicular block, only one fascicle of the left bundle branch is supplying electrical current to the bulk of both ventricles. The EKG findings include a combination of features of both hemiblock and right bundle branch block.

Criteria for Bifascicular Block

The features of right bundle branch block combined with left anterior hemiblock are as follows:

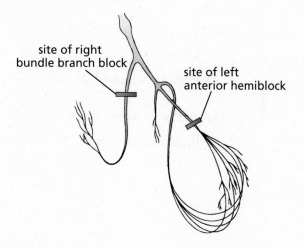

site of right
bundle branch block

site of left
anterior hemiblock

Right Bundle Branch Block

- QRS wider than 0.12 seconds
- RSR′ in V1 and V2.

Left Anterior Hemiblock

- Left axis deviation between −30° and +90°.

The features of right bundle branch block combined with left posterior hemiblock are as follows:

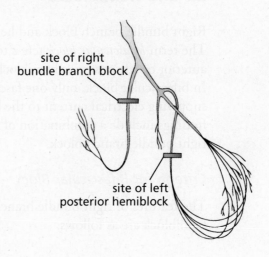

site of right
bundle branch block

site of left
posterior hemiblock

Right Bundle Branch Block

- QRS wider than 0.12 seconds
- RSR′ in V1 and V2.

Left Posterior Hemiblock

- Right axis deviation.

Can you identify a bifascicular block on this EKG?

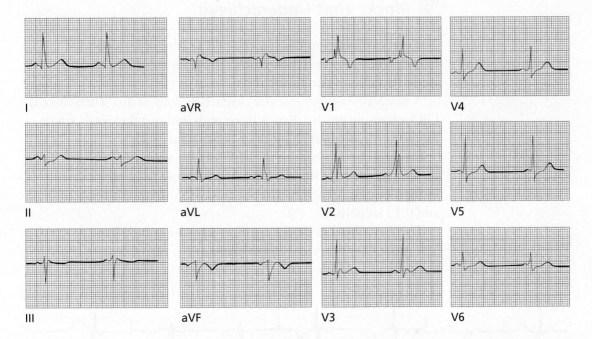

This is an example of right bundle branch block combined with left anterior hemiblock. Note the widened QRS complex and rabbit ears in leads V1 and V2, characteristic of right bundle branch block, and the left axis deviation in the limb leads (the QRS complex is predominantly positive in lead I and negative in leads aVF and II) that suggests left anterior hemiblock.

Blocks That Underachieve

Not every conduction block meets all the criteria for a bundle branch block or bifascicular block. These are extremely common and generally fall into two types:

A *nonspecific intraventricular conduction delay* occurs when there is QRS widening greater than 0.10 seconds without the usual criteria for either bundle branch block or bifascicular block.

An *incomplete bundle branch block* occurs when the EKG tracing shows a left or right bundle branch appearance (*e.g.*, rabbit ears in V1 in right bundle branch block) but the QRS duration is between 0.10 and 0.12 seconds.

These conduction blocks are caused by the same disease processes that cause the other conduction blocks.

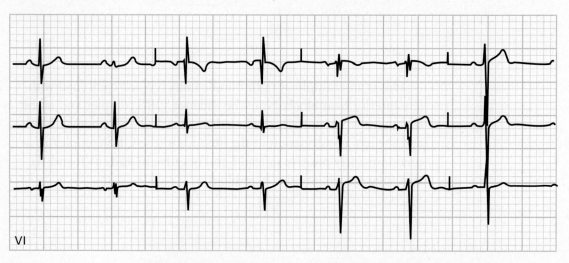

VI

Incomplete right bundle branch block; the QRS complex is not widened, but note the classic rabbit ears configuration in V1.

The Ultimate in Playing With Blocks: Combining AV Blocks, Right Bundle Branch Block, and Hemiblocks

Right bundle branch block, hemiblocks, and bifascicular blocks can also occur in combination with AV blocks. (Are you sure you're ready for this?) Take a look at the following EKG and see if you can identify the different conduction blocks that are present. An orderly approach is essential.

1. Is there any AV block? Look at the relationship between the P waves and QRS complexes.

2. Is there any bundle branch block? Look in the precordial leads for wide QRS complexes with their distinctive configurations; are there any ST segment and T wave changes?

3. Is there any hemiblock? Look for axis deviation.

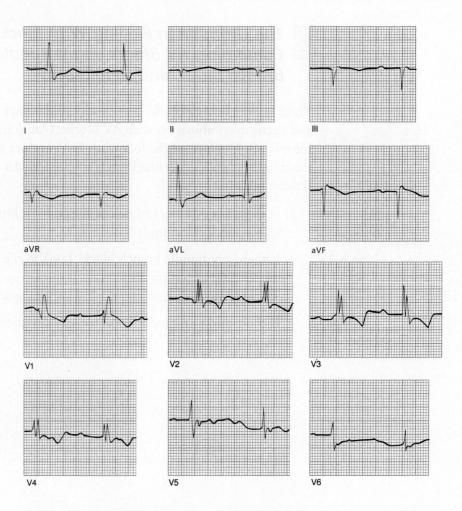

This EKG shows

1. first-degree AV block (the PR interval exceeds 0.20 seconds)

2. right bundle branch block (there are wide QRS complexes with rabbit ears in leads V1 through V4)

3. left anterior hemiblock (left axis deviation is present).

Pacemakers

Many pacemakers, both temporary and permanent, are inserted every year, and in the right circumstances they can relieve symptoms of inadequate cardiac output and prevent sudden death from complete conduction block or a tachyarrhythmia. Clinical evidence strongly supports their use in patients with

- third-degree (complete) AV block

- a lesser degree of AV block or bradycardia *(e.g.,* sick sinus syndrome) if the patient is symptomatic (especially in atrial fibrillation)

- the sudden development of various combinations of AV block and bundle branch block in patients who are in the throes of an acute myocardial infarction (this situation usually only requires a temporary pacemaker that can be removed after the acute incident has resolved)

- recurrent tachycardias that can be overdriven and thereby terminated by pacemaker activity.

Pacemakers are nothing more than a power source controlled by a microchip and connected to electrodes. The power source is usually placed subcutaneously, and the electrodes are threaded into the right atrium and right ventricle through veins that drain to the heart. Pacemakers provide an alternate source of electrical stimulation for a heart whose own intrinsic source of electricity (the sinus node) or whose ability to conduct electrical current is impaired.

Pacemaker technology has accelerated dramatically in recent years. Whereas early pacemakers were capable of firing only at a single predetermined rate *(fixed rate pacemakers)* no matter what the heart itself was doing, today's pacemakers are responsive to the moment-to-moment needs of the heart. They are programmable in terms of sensitivity, rate of firing, refractory period, and so on. The present generation of pacemakers can even increase the heart rate in response to motion or increased respirations for those patients who cannot increase their own heart rate appropriately during activity, because of either disease of the sinus node or the effects of medications.

The most popular pacemaker today is a *demand pacemaker*. A demand pacemaker fires only when the patient's own intrinsic heart rate falls below a threshold level. For example, a demand pacemaker set at 60 beats per minute will remain silent as long as the patient's heart rate remains above 60 beats per minute. As soon as there is a pause between beats that would translate into a rate below 60, the pacemaker will fire.

Pacemaker electrodes can be placed in the atrium or ventricle alone (single-chamber pacemakers) or, more commonly, in both chambers (dual-chamber pacemakers). Dual-chamber pacemakers are also called A-V sequential pacemakers. In patients with third-degree heart block with an origin near the AV node, atrial pacemakers would be useless because their electrical impulses would fail to penetrate into the ventricles; instead, ventricular or A-V sequential pacemakers need to be used.

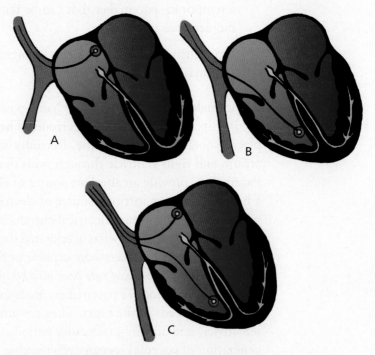

(*A*) Site of atrial pacemaker implantation. (*B*) Ventricular pacemaker. (*C*) Sequential pacemaker with atrial and ventricular leads.

When a pacemaker fires, a small spike can be seen on the EKG. With a ventricular pacemaker, the ensuing QRS complex will be wide and bizarre, just like a PVC. Because the electrodes are located in the right ventricle, the right ventricle will contract first and then the left ventricle. This generates a pattern identical to left bundle branch block, with delayed left ventricular activation. A retrograde P wave may or may not be seen.

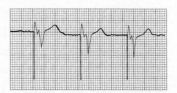

EKG from a patient with a ventricular pacemaker.

An atrial pacemaker will generate a spike followed by a P wave and a normal QRS complex.

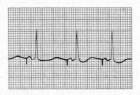

EKG from a patient with an atrial pacemaker.

With a sequential pacemaker, two spikes will be seen, one preceding a P wave and one preceding a wide, bizarre QRS complex.

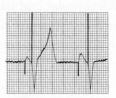

EKG from a patient with a sequential pacemaker.

When used appropriately, pacemakers save lives. They can, however, be very dangerous even in the best of circumstances. The pacemaker spike itself always has the potential to induce a serious arrhythmia. For example, if a ventricular pacemaker should happen to fire mistakenly during the vulnerable period of ventricular repolarization (remember the R-on-T phenomenon?), ventricular tachycardia can be induced. Fortunately, advancements in pacemaker design have made this a rare occurrence as long as the electrodes maintain good contact with the heart.

Patients with impaired left ventricular function or congestive heart failure may not always benefit from a pacemaker inserted in the right ventricle (depicted in figures *B* and *C* on page 196). Indeed, such a pacemaker may actually precipitate an episode of heart failure by overriding effective intrinsic electrical conduction and worsening ventricular contractile function. Thus, a newer pacing option has been introduced for such patients in which a third electrode is threaded into the coronary sinus from the right atrium and passed into the lateral veins of the left ventricle where *epicardial* pacing enhances left ventricular conduction and reduces the symptoms of heart failure (see the following figure).

Another group of patients who may benefit from this type of pacemaker are those with left bundle branch block, which causes dysynchrony of the right ventricular and left ventricular contractions and in this way may impair ventricular function. The left ventricular pacemaker can correct this faulty timing and again improve the patient's clinical situation. This so-called *cardiac resynchronization therapy* (CRT) has been shown to reduce rates of hospitalization and death in patients with class II and class III heart failure. CRT only benefits patients whose heart failure is associated with a wide QRS complex and left ventricular systolic dysfunction. Interestingly, however, the degree to which biventricular pacing narrows the QRS complex does not correlate with therapeutic benefit.

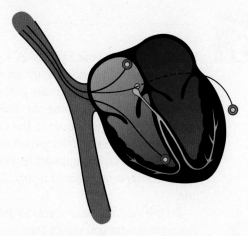

Site of an epicardial pacemaker.

In some patients, pacemaker spikes can be difficult to see on a standard EKG because their amplitude may be less than 1 mV. If you are examining an EKG from a patient unknown to you that demonstrates wide QRS complexes and left axis deviation, you must always suspect the presence of a pacemaker even if the tiny pacemaker spikes cannot be seen. Obviously, examination of the patient or—if the patient is lucid—a simple question or two will reveal the presence or absence of an electrical pacemaker.

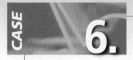

CASE

6.

Sally M. works at your hospital as a volunteer. One day she is instructed to take some intravenous solutions from the pharmacy in the hospital basement to the intensive care unit on the third floor. At the same time, you just happen to be standing at the third floor elevator, waiting impatiently for a ride down to the cafeteria. When the elevator door opens, you find Sally collapsed on the floor. A quick purview of her vital signs reveals that she appears hemodynamically stable. You grab a gurney that is conveniently parked nearby and rush her into the intensive care unit.

On the way to the unit you try talking to her. She is confused and disoriented, and you notice that she has been incontinent. In the intensive care unit (ICU), this rhythm strip is obtained:

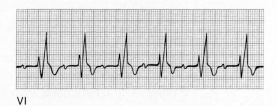

VI

Does this rhythm strip tell you what happened to Sally on the elevator?

In a word, no. The rhythm strip reveals a modest sinus tachycardia, first-degree AV block, and the rabbit ears of right bundle branch block. Nothing here can account for her collapse. Had you found significant bradycardia, a ventricular arrhythmia, or an advanced degree of heart block, you would certainly have cause to suspect the presence of Stokes-Adams syncope, that is, a sudden faint from inadequate cardiac output. The period of disorientation following her collapse is also not typical of Stokes-Adams syncope but is typical of the postictal state seen after a seizure.

About 15 minutes after her collapse, Sally's mental state has returned to normal, and she is anxious to return to work. You are able to persuade her that a short stay in the ICU for observation would be a good idea. Continual cardiac monitoring reveals no significant arrhythmias or conduction blocks, but a magnetic resonance imaging (MRI) of her head does reveal a probable meningioma. It is likely, therefore, that Sally did suffer a seizure caused by an expanding (but fortunately not malignant) brain lesion. The meningioma is excised without complication, and several months later, you see Sally happily plying her trade once again, a joyful reminder to all that performing a service for others is the surest way to achieve true satisfaction in life.

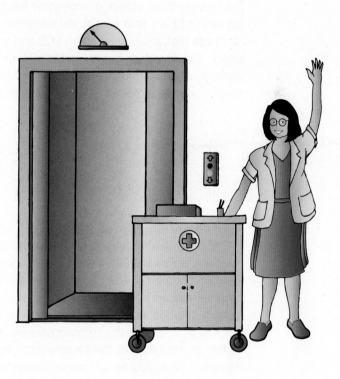

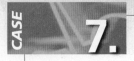

CASE 7.

Jonathan N., dressed in a magnificent three-piece bespoke suit and wearing hand-sewn shoes whose cost could fund an overseas medical clinic for a month, is the chief executive officer of a large investment firm, a position he describes as "more stressful than anything you, my friend, could ever imagine." He is new to your practice and tells you that he has recently been suffering from some exertional shortness of breath but doesn't have time for "all the nonsense of a history and physical." He insists that you simply run an EKG and tell him if he is having a heart attack. Taking a deep breath and trying not to roll your eyes too obviously, you hook him up to your EKG machine. The 12-lead EKG does not show any acute ischemia, but lead V1 does show this:

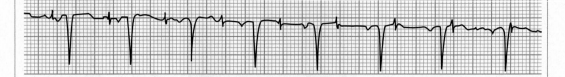

What do you see, what do you infer, and what do you do?

The most striking finding is the procession of pacemaker spikes marching across the EKG bearing no relation whatsoever to the P waves and QRS complexes. The pacemaker is failing to capture the heart. You can infer a heart history that required the pacemaker in the first place. Because the rate and rhythm appears to be otherwise well maintained, it is not at all clear that this consummate executive's shortness of breath is related to the failure of the pacemaker to adequately capture and drive the heart. What you do, of course, is now insist on a careful history and physical to guide your next move (You will not be not surprised to learn that he has a history of high degrees of AV block and a prior myocardial infarction).

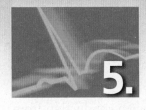

5. Preexcitation Syndromes

In this chapter you will learn:

1 | what happens when electrical current is conducted to the ventricles more rapidly than usual

2 | what an accessory pathway is

3 | that Wolff-Parkinson-White and Lown-Ganong-Levine are not the names of law firms

4 | why accessory pathways predispose to arrhythmias

5 | about the case of Winston T., a *preexcitable* personality.

What Is Preexcitation?

In the last chapter, we discussed what happens when conduction from the atria to the ventricles is delayed or blocked. This chapter presents the other side of the coin: what happens when the electrical current is conducted to the ventricles *more quickly than usual.*

How can such a thing happen?

With normal conduction, the major delay between the atria and the ventricles is in the atrioventricular (AV) node, where the wave of depolarization is held up for about 0.1 second, long enough for the atria to contract and empty their content of circulating blood into the ventricles. In the *preexcitation syndromes*, there are *accessory pathways* by which the current can bypass the AV node and thus arrive at the ventricles ahead of time.

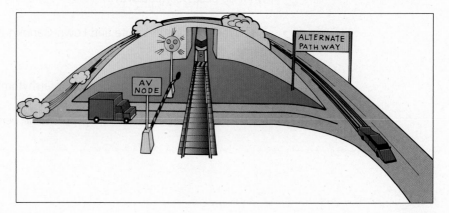

A number of different accessory pathways have been discovered. Probably fewer than 1% of individuals possess one of these pathways. There is a decided male preponderance. Accessory pathways may occur in normal healthy hearts as an isolated finding, or they may occur in conjunction with mitral valve prolapse, hypertrophic cardiomyopathies, and various congenital disorders.

There are two major preexcitation syndromes: *Wolff-Parkinson-White (WPW) syndrome* and *Lown-Ganong-Levine (LGL) syndrome*. They are both easily diagnosed on the EKG. In both syndromes, the accessory conduction pathways act as short circuits, allowing the atrial wave of depolarization to bypass the AV node and activate the ventricles prematurely.

Wolff-Parkinson-White Syndrome

In WPW syndrome, the bypass pathway has been named the *bundle of Kent*. It is a discrete aberrant conducting pathway that connects the atria and ventricles. It can be left sided (connecting the left atrium and left ventricle) or right sided (connecting the right atrium and right ventricle).

Premature ventricular depolarization through the bundle of Kent causes two things to happen on the EKG:

1. The PR interval, representing the time from the start of atrial depolarization to the start of ventricular depolarization, is shortened. The criterion for diagnosis is a *PR interval less than 0.12 seconds.*

2. The QRS complex is widened to more than 0.1 second. Unlike bundle branch block, in which the QRS complex is widened because of *delayed* ventricular activation, in WPW it is widened because of *premature* activation. The QRS complex in WPW actually represents a fusion beat: most of the ventricular myocardium is activated through the normal conduction pathways, but a small region is depolarized early through the bundle of Kent. This small region of myocardium that is depolarized early gives the QRS complex a characteristic slurred initial upstroke called a *delta wave*. A true delta wave may be seen in only a few leads, so scan the entire EKG.

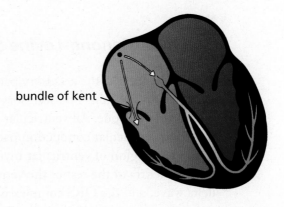

bundle of kent

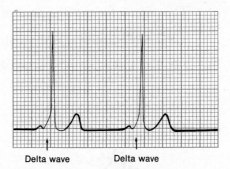

Delta wave   Delta wave

WPW syndrome. Current is held up by the normal delay at the AV node but races unimpeded down the bundle of Kent. The EKG shows the short PR interval and delta wave.

Lown-Ganong-Levine Syndrome

In LGL syndrome, the accessory pathway (called James fiber) is effectively *intranodal*. The accessory pathway bypasses the delay within the AV node. All ventricular conduction occurs through the usual ventricular conduction pathways; unlike WPW, there is no small region of ventricular myocardium that is depolarized independently of the rest of the ventricles. Therefore, there is no delta wave, and the QRS complex is not widened. The only electrical manifestation of LGL is a shortening of the PR interval as a result of the accessory pathway bypassing the delay within the AV node. The criteria for the diagnosis of LGL are as follows:

- The PR interval is shortened to less than 0.12 seconds.

- The QRS complex is not widened.

- There is no delta wave.

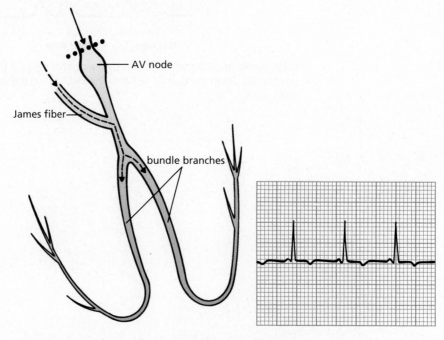

In LGL syndrome, the PR interval is short, but there is no delta wave.

Associated Arrhythmias

In many individuals with WPW or LGL, preexcitation poses few, if any, clinical problems. However, preexcitation does predispose to various tachyarrhythmias. This predisposition has been most clearly documented in WPW, where it is estimated that 50% to 70% of individuals experience at least one supraventricular arrhythmia.

The two tachyarrhythmias most often seen in WPW are *paroxysmal supraventricular tachycardia (PSVT)* and *atrial fibrillation.*

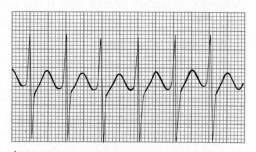

A

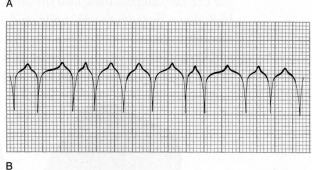

B

(*A*) Paroxysmal supraventricular tachycardia. (*B*) Atrial fibrillation.

Paroxysmal Supraventricular Tachycardia in WPW

In normal hearts, PSVT usually arises through a reentrant mechanism. The same is true in WPW. In fact, the presence of an accessory bundle—an alternate pathway of conduction—is the *perfect* substrate for reentry. Here is how it works.

We have already seen how, in WPW, a normal beat generates a QRS complex that is a fusion of two waves, one conducted through the bundle of Kent (the delta wave) and one through the AV node and along the normal pathway of conduction. Although the bundle of Kent usually conducts current faster than the AV node, it also tends to have a longer refractory period once it has been depolarized. What happens, then, if a normal sinus impulse is followed abruptly by a premature atrial beat? This premature beat will be conducted normally through the AV node, but the bundle of Kent may still be refractory, blocking conduction through the alternate route. The wave of depolarization will then move through the AV node and into the bundle branches and ventricular myocardium. By the time it encounters the bundle of Kent on the ventricular side, it may no longer be refractory, and the current can pass back into the atria. It is then free to pass right back down through the AV node, and a self-sustaining, revolving reentrant mechanism has been established. The result is PSVT. The QRS complex during the arrhythmia is narrow because ventricular depolarization occurs through the normal bundle branches.

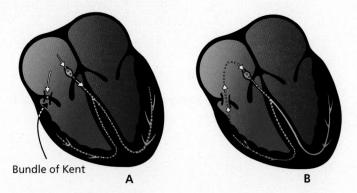

Bundle of Kent

A   **B**

The formation of a reentry circuit in WPW syndrome. A premature atrial beat sends current down the normal conduction pathways but not through the refractory bundle of Kent (*A*). Current then circles back through the bundle of Kent, which is no longer refractory to conduction, to form a complete reentrant circuit (*B*).

Less commonly, the reentrant mechanism circles the other way; that is, down the bundle of Kent and back up through the AV node. The result, again, is PSVT, but now the QRS complex is wide and bizarre because ventricular depolarization does not occur along the normal bundle branches. This arrhythmia may be indistinguishable from ventricular tachycardia on the EKG.

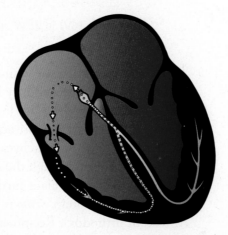

A second type of reentry circuit in WPW syndrome. Current moves antegrade down the bundle of Kent and then retrograde through the AV node, establishing an independent revolving circuit.

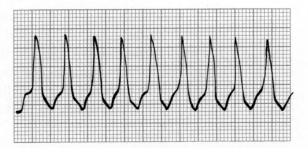

Wide-complex PSVT in WPW syndrome.

You may recall that the "usual" form of PSVT in normal hearts is most often caused by a reentry loop within the AV node. Here, in WPW, because the reentrant loop reciprocates between the atria and ventricles, the PSVT is more accurately termed **AV reciprocating tachycardia.** When the tachycardia activates the ventricles in an antegrade manner through the AV node, generating a narrow QRS complex, the arrhythmia is further subcategorized as an **orthodromic tachycardia** (the prefix *ortho* is intended to convey the meaning of correct, or orthodox). Reciprocating tachycardias that activate the ventricles through the accessory pathway, generating a wide QRS complex, are subcategorized as **antidromic tachycardia.**

In 10% to 15% of patients with WPW, there is more than one accessory pathway, permitting the formation of multiple reentry loops as the current passes up and down through the different Kent bundles and the AV node.

Atrial Fibrillation in WPW

Atrial fibrillation, the other arrhythmia commonly seen in WPW, can be particularly devastating. The bundle of Kent can act as a free conduit for the chaotic atrial activity. Without the AV node to act as a barrier between the atria and ventricles, ventricular rates can rise as high as 300 beats per minute. The precise rate will depend on the refractory period of the bundle of Kent. This rapid atrial fibrillation has been known to induce ventricular fibrillation, a lethal arrhythmia. Fortunately, this lethal form of atrial fibrillation is rare in WPW, but it must be considered a diagnostic possibility in patients who have been resuscitated from an episode of sudden death or syncope and are found to have preexcitation on their cardiograms.

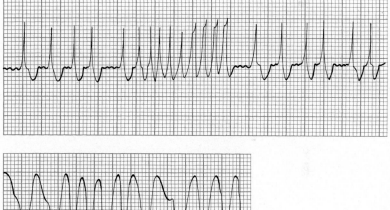

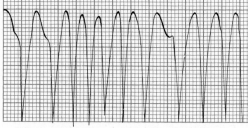

Two examples of atrial fibrillation in WPW syndrome. The ventricular rate is extremely fast.

Mapping the aberrant pathways in patients with WPW can be accomplished during EPS, and has become routine in affected patients who are symptomatic or have documented arrhythmias.

During the mapping procedure, the atrial–ventricular connection can be ablated, thereby resolving the problem.

> Patients with WPW do have an increased risk of sudden death, but this is only very rarely the presenting feature, allowing time for successful clinical intervention before an episode of sudden death can occur. The overall prognosis today for patients with WPW is excellent.

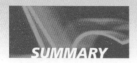

SUMMARY

Preexcitation

The diagnosis of preexcitation is made by looking for a short PR interval.

Criteria for WPW Syndrome

1. PR interval less than 0.12 seconds

2. Wide QRS complexes

3. Delta wave seen in some leads.

Criteria for LGL Syndrome

1. PR interval less than 0.12 seconds

2. Normal QRS width

3. No delta wave.

Arrhythmias commonly seen include the following:

1. Paroxysmal supraventricular tachycardia—narrow QRS complexes are more common than wide ones.

2. Atrial fibrillation—can be very rapid and rarely can lead to ventricular fibrillation.

> Because the presence of an accessory pathway in WPW alters the vectors of current flow to at least some degree, you cannot assess axis or amplitude with any precision, and hence any attempt to determine the presence of ventricular hypertrophy or bundle branch block is bound to be unreliable.

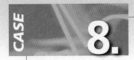

CASE 8.

Winston T., a young biochemical engineer, is brought to the emergency room by his wife. During dinner, he became light-headed and nauseated (not an uncommon event during dinner at the Winston household, but the severity of the symptoms prompted concern).

In the emergency room, Winston denies any chest pain or shortness of breath.

The medical student who is the first to examine him has seen just enough patients to feel overconfident in his diagnostic abilities. Tired and overworked, he listens to Winston's story and is ready to send Winston home with a diagnosis of food poisoning when an astute nurse takes the trouble to put a hand on Winston's pulse and discovers it is extremely rapid. An EKG reveals:

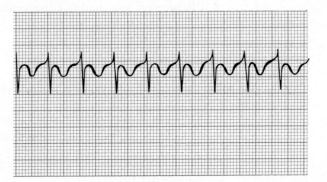

Distraught by his carelessness, the medical student becomes somewhat pallid himself. The emergency room doctor takes over, glances at the rhythm strip and immediately orders a dose of intravenous adenosine. The tachycardia breaks at once, and the new rhythm strip looks like this:

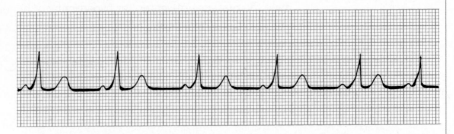

Can you match the emergency room doctor's heady acumen with erudition of your own and figure out exactly what has happened?

Winston has WPW syndrome. This is readily apparent from the second EKG, which reveals the characteristic short PR interval, delta wave, and prolonged QRS complex. The initial strip shows the typical narrow QRS complex PSVT that can occur in these individuals. The rapid tachycardia was responsible for Winston's symptoms, not his undercooked Cornish game hen.

Intravenous adenosine, a potent AV node blocking agent with a half-life of less than 10 seconds, is extremely effective at breaking reentrant tachycardias that involve the AV node. This was Winston's first attack, and because most patients with WPW have only infrequent episodes of tachycardia, chronic antiarrhythmic therapy is not indicated at this time.

As for what became of the medical student, he learned from his humiliating experience and went on to become a model of thoroughness and efficiency, eventually graduating at the top of his class. He also has never forgotten the first rule of medicine: **always take the vital signs.** There is good reason why they are called "vital."

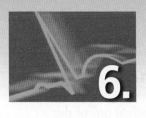

6. Myocardial Ischemia and Infarction

In this chapter you will learn:

1 | the three things that happen to the EKG during a myocardial infarction (T wave peaking and inversion, ST segment elevation, and the appearance of new Q waves)

2 | how to distinguish normal Q waves from the Q waves of infarction

3 | how the EKG can localize an infarct to a particular region of the heart

4 | the difference between Q wave and non–Q wave infarctions

5 | how the EKG changes during an attack of angina (ST segment depression and T wave inversion)

6 | how to distinguish typical angina from Prinzmetal's (vasospastic) angina on the EKG

7 | the value of stress testing in diagnosing coronary artery disease

8 | about the case of Joan L., a woman with an acute infarction and a number of complications requiring your acute attention.

What Is a Myocardial Infarction?

A myocardial infarction, or "heart attack," occurs when one of the coronary arteries becomes totally occluded. The region of myocardium supplied by that particular coronary artery loses its blood supply and, deprived of oxygen and other nutrients, dies. The underlying pathogenesis in almost all cases is progressive narrowing of the coronary arteries by atherosclerosis. The sudden, total occlusion that precipitates infarction is usually due to superimposed thrombosis or coronary artery spasm.

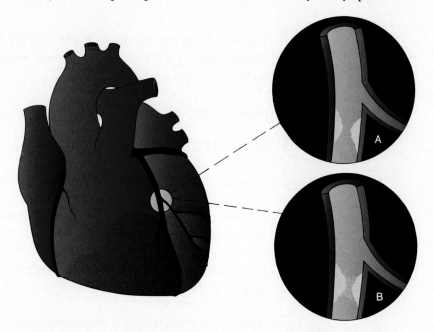

Occlusion of a coronary artery can lead to infarction of the region of myocardium that is dependent on that artery for its blood supply.
(*A*) The coronary artery is gradually narrowed by atherosclerotic plaque.
(*B*) Infarction can be caused by an acute thrombus superimposed on the underlying plaque.

How to Diagnose a Myocardial Infarction

There are three components to the diagnosis of a myocardial infarction: (1) history and physical examination; (2) cardiac enzyme determinations; and (3) the EKG.

History and Physical Examination. When a patient presents with the typical features of infarction—prolonged, crushing substernal chest pain radiating to the jaw, shoulders, or left arm, associated with nausea, diaphoresis, and shortness of breath—there can be little doubt about the diagnosis. However, many patients, especially those with diabetes mellitus and elderly individuals, may not manifest all of these symptoms. It is estimated that up to one-third of myocardial infarctions are "silent"; that is, they are not associated with any overt clinical manifestations at all.

Cardiac Enzymes. Dying myocardial cells leak their internal contents into the bloodstream. Elevated blood levels of *creatine kinase* (CK), particularly the MB isoenzyme, are strongly indicative of an infarction and have long been a mainstay of diagnosis. However, for several reasons, elevated levels of the cardiac *troponin* enzyme have, if not supplanted CK levels, at least begun to occupy a more prominent role in the laboratory diagnosis of myocardial infarction. Troponin enzyme determinations (either for troponin I or troponin T), especially the newer high-sensitivity assays, are very sensitive and specific for myocardial infarction. Troponin levels rise earlier than the CK-MB isoenzyme (within 2 to 3 hours) and may stay elevated for several days. CK levels do not usually rise until 6 hours after an infarction and return to normal within 48 hours.

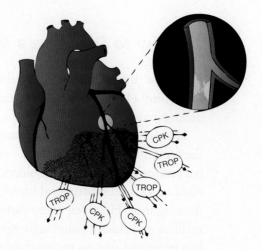

Intracellular enzymes are released by the dying myocardial cells after complete coronary occlusion resulting in acute infarction.

The EKG. In most infarctions, the EKG will reveal the correct diagnosis. Characteristic electrocardiographic changes accompany myocardial infarction, and the earliest changes occur almost at once with the onset of myocardial compromise. An EKG should be performed immediately on anyone in whom an infarction is even remotely suspected. However, the initial EKG may not always be diagnostic, and the evolution of electrocardiographic changes varies from person to person; therefore, it is necessary to obtain serial cardiograms once the patient is admitted to the hospital.

During an acute myocardial infarction, the EKG evolves through three stages:

1. T wave peaking followed by T wave inversion (*A* and *B*, below)

2. ST segment elevation (*C*)

3. Appearance of new Q waves (*D*).

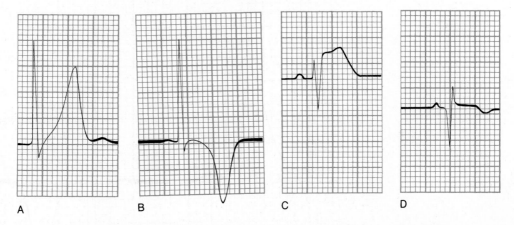

(*A*) T wave peaking, (*B*) T wave inversion, (*C*) ST segment elevation, (*D*) formation of a new Q wave.

Although the EKG does typically evolve through these three stages during an acute infarction, any one of these changes may be present without any of the others. Thus, for example, it is not at all unusual to see ST segment elevation without T wave inversion. In addition, many myocardial infarctions do *not* generate Q waves (to be discussed later in this chapter). Nevertheless, learn to recognize each of these three changes, keep your suspicion of myocardial infarction high, and you will almost never go wrong.

The T Wave

With the onset of infarction, the T waves become tall and narrow, a phenomenon called *peaking*. These peaked T waves are often referred to as *hyperacute T waves*. Shortly afterward, usually a few hours later, the T waves invert.

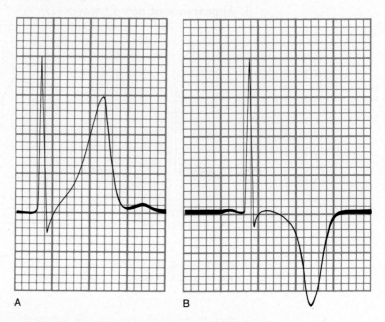

(A) T wave peaking in a patient undergoing acute infarction. (B) The same lead in a patient 2 hours later shows T wave inversion.

These T wave changes reflect myocardial *ischemia,* the lack of adequate blood flow to the myocardium.

Ischemia is potentially reversible: if blood flow is restored or the oxygen demands of the heart are eased, the T waves will revert to normal. On the other hand, if actual myocardial cell death (true infarction) has occurred, T wave inversion will persist for months to years.

T wave inversion by itself is indicative only of ischemia and is not diagnostic of myocardial infarction.

T wave inversion is a very nonspecific finding. Many things can cause a T wave to flip; for example, we have already seen that both bundle branch block and ventricular hypertrophy with repolarization abnormalities are associated with T wave inversion.

One helpful diagnostic feature is that the T waves of myocardial ischemia are inverted *symmetrically*, whereas in most other circumstances they are asymmetric, with a gentle downslope and rapid upslope.

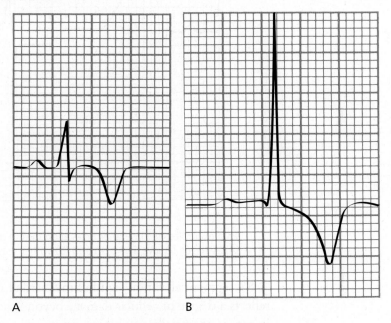

A   B

(*A*) The symmetric T wave inversion in a patient with ischemia.
(*B*) An example of asymmetric T wave inversion in a patient with left ventricular hypertrophy and repolarization abnormalities.

In patients whose T waves are already inverted, ischemia may cause them to revert to normal, a phenomenon called *pseudonormalization*. Recognition of pseudonormalization requires comparing the current EKG with a previous tracing.

The ST Segment

ST segment elevation is the second change that occurs acutely in the evolution of an infarction.

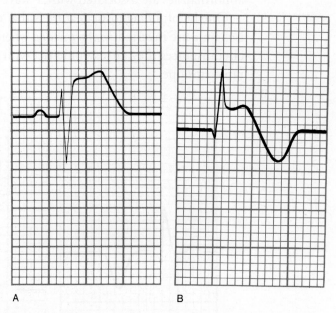

A   B

Two examples of ST segment elevation during an acute infarction:
(*A*) Without T wave inversion and (*B*) with T wave inversion.

ST segment elevation signifies myocardial *injury*. Injury probably reflects a degree of cellular damage beyond that of mere ischemia, but it, too, is potentially reversible, and in some cases, the ST segments may rapidly return to normal. In most instances, however, ST segment elevation is a reliable sign that true infarction has occurred and that the complete electrocardiographic picture of infarction will evolve unless there is immediate and aggressive therapeutic intervention.

Even in the setting of a true infarction, the ST segments usually return to baseline within a few hours. Persistent ST segment elevation often indicates the formation of a *ventricular aneurysm,* a weakening and bulging of the ventricular wall.

Like T wave inversion, ST segment elevation can be seen in a number of other conditions in addition to an evolving myocardial infarction—the most common of these are listed on page 248 and are addressed in Chapter 7. There is even a type of ST segment elevation that can be seen in normal hearts. This phenomenon has been referred to as *early repolarization* (actually a physiologic misnomer) or *J point elevation* (a much better term). The *J point*, or *junction point*, is the place where the ST segment takes off from the QRS complex.

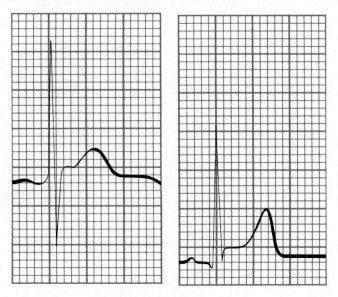

Two examples of J point elevation.

J point elevation is very common in young, healthy individuals. The ST segment usually returns to baseline with exercise. J point elevation has long been thought to have no pathologic implications. However, some research has reported a slightly increased risk of death from cardiac causes in patients with J point elevation in the inferior leads.

How can the ST segment elevation of myocardial injury be distinguished from that of J point elevation? With myocardial injury, the elevated ST segment has a distinctive configuration. It is bowed upward and tends to merge imperceptibly with the T wave. In J point elevation, the T wave maintains its independent waveform.

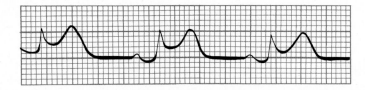

ST segment elevation during an infarction. Note how the ST segment and T wave merge into each other without a clear demarcation between them.

Q Waves

The appearance of new Q waves indicates that irreversible myocardial cell death has occurred. The presence of Q waves is diagnostic of myocardial infarction.

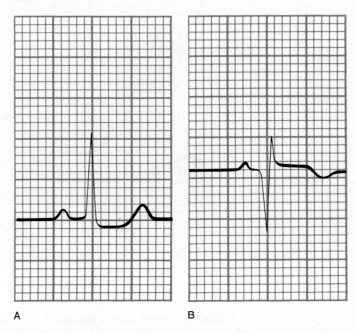

A   B

(A) Lead III in a healthy patient. (B) The same lead in the same patient 2 weeks after undergoing an inferior myocardial infarction. Note the deep Q wave.

Q waves usually appear within several hours of the onset of infarction, but in some patients they may take several days to evolve. The ST segment usually has returned to baseline by the time Q waves have appeared. Q waves usually persist for the lifetime of the patient.

Why Q Waves Form

The genesis of Q waves as a sign of infarction is easy to understand. When a region of myocardium dies, it becomes electrically silent—it is no longer able to conduct an electrical current. As a result, all of the electrical forces of the heart will be directed *away* from the area of infarction. An electrode overlying the infarct will therefore record a deep negative deflection, a Q wave.

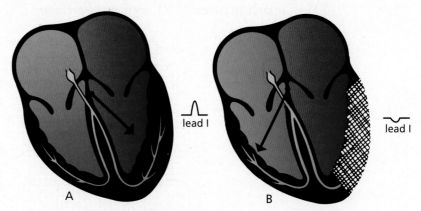

(*A*) Normal left ventricular depolarization with the arrow showing the electrical axis. Note the tall R wave in lead I. (*B*) The lateral wall of the left ventricle has infarcted and, as a result, is now electrically silent. The electrical axis therefore shifts rightward, away from lead I, which now shows a negative deflection (Q wave).

Reciprocal Changes

Other leads, located some distance from the site of infarction, will see an apparent *increase* in the electrical forces moving toward them. They will record tall positive R waves.

These opposing changes seen by distant leads are called *reciprocal changes*. The concept of reciprocity applies not only to Q waves but also to ST segment and T wave changes. Thus, a lead distant from an infarct may record ST segment *depression*.

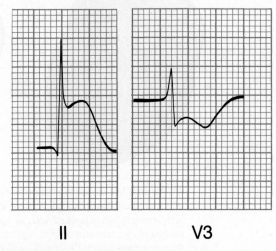

II   V3

Reciprocal changes in an inferior infarction. The acute ST elevation and T wave peaking in lead II is echoed by the ST depression and T wave inversion in lead V3.

Normal Versus Pathologic Q Waves

Small Q waves can be seen in the left lateral leads (I, aVL, V5, and V6) and occasionally in the inferior leads (especially II and III) of perfectly normal hearts. These Q waves are caused by the early left-to-right depolarization of the interventricular septum.

Pathologic Q waves signifying infarction are *wider* and *deeper*. They are often referred to as *significant Q waves*. The criteria for significance are the following:

1. The Q wave must be greater than 0.04 seconds in duration.

2. The depth of the Q wave must be at least one-third the height of the R wave in the same QRS complex.

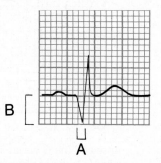

An example of a significant Q wave. Its width (*A*) exceeds 0.04 seconds, and its depth (*B*) exceeds one-third that of the R wave.

Note: Because lead aVR occupies a unique position on the frontal plane, it normally has a very deep Q wave. Lead aVR should not be considered when assessing possible infarction.

Are the following Q waves significant?

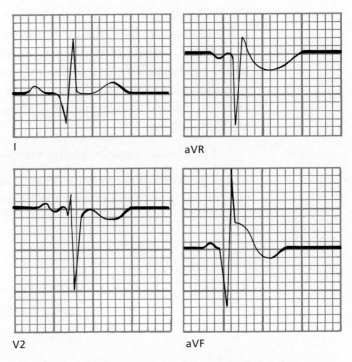

Answers: The Q waves in leads I and aVF are significant. The Q wave in lead V2 is too shallow and narrow to qualify (don't confuse the tiny Q wave with the large S wave). The Q wave in lead aVR is immense, but Q waves in aVR are never significant!

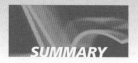

SUMMARY   The EKG Changes of an Evolving Myocardial Infarction

1. Acutely, the T wave peaks and then inverts. T wave changes reflect myocardial ischemia. If true infarction occurs, the T wave remains inverted for months to years.

2. Acutely, the ST segment elevates and merges with the T wave. ST segment elevation reflects myocardial injury. If infarction occurs, the ST segment usually returns to baseline within a few hours.

3. New Q waves appear within hours to days. They signify myocardial infarction. In most cases, they persist for the lifetime of the patient.

The term *acute coronary syndrome* is used to refer to individuals with unstable coronary disease or an evolving infarction in whom emergent therapy can prevent additional damage and possibly even be lifesaving. It is critical to recognize an evolving myocardial infarction as early as possible because therapy is widely available that—delivered within the first few hours after the onset of an infarction—can prevent the completion of the infarct and improve survival. Thrombolytic agents and direct plasminogen activators can lyse a clot within the coronary arteries and restore blood flow before myocardial death has occurred. In hospitals with catheterization and angioplasty capabilities, emergency angioplasty within the first 6 hours of the onset of infarction offers superior survival to thrombolysis alone, both acutely and in long-term follow-up.

Once angioplasty has been successfully carried out, the placement of stents coated with cytotoxic drugs to prevent reocclusion (usually a result of cell proliferation) at the site of the original lesion has reduced the rate of restenosis from about one-third of patients undergoing angioplasty to virtually none. The administration of both oral and intravenous platelet-inhibiting agents (glycoprotein IIb/IIIa inhibitors) has further improved patient outcome.

Whichever intervention is available or chosen, the key to successful therapy is timing: you must intervene quickly. The recognition of the acute changes of a myocardial infarction on the EKG is a critical diagnostic skill that can save lives.

Localizing the Infarct

The region of myocardium that undergoes infarction depends on which coronary artery becomes occluded and the extent of collateral blood flow. There are two major systems of blood supply to the myocardium, one supplying the right side of the heart and one supplying the left side.

The *right coronary artery* runs between the right atrium and right ventricle and then swings around to the posterior surface of the heart. In most individuals, it gives off a descending branch that supplies the atrioventricular (AV) node.

The *left main artery* divides into a *left anterior descending (LAD) artery* and a *left circumflex artery*. The LAD supplies the anterior wall of the heart and most of the interventricular septum. The circumflex artery runs between the left atrium and left ventricle and supplies the lateral wall of the left ventricle. In about 10% of the population, it gives off the branch that supplies the AV node.

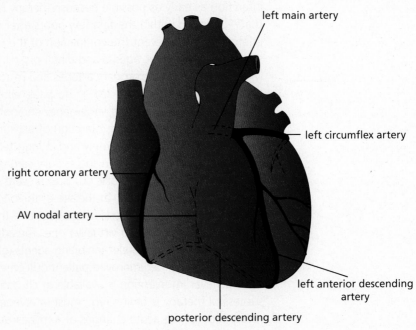

The main coronary arteries.

Localization of an infarct is important because the prognostic and therapeutic implications are in part determined by which area of the heart is affected.

Infarctions can be grouped into several general anatomic categories. These categories include inferior, lateral, anterior, and posterior infarctions. Combinations can also be seen, such as anterolateral and inferoposterior infarctions.

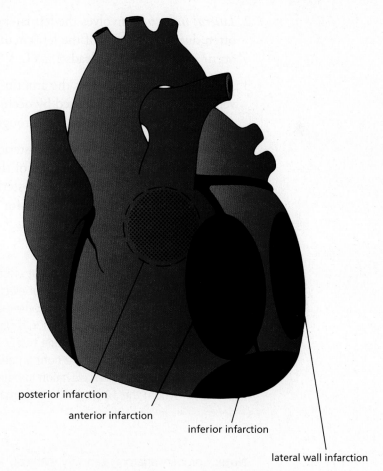

posterior infarction

anterior infarction

inferior infarction

lateral wall infarction

The four basic anatomic sites of myocardial infarction.

Almost all myocardial infarctions involve the left ventricle. This should not be surprising because the left ventricle is the most muscular chamber and is called on to do the most work. It is therefore most vulnerable to a compromised blood supply.

The characteristic electrocardiographic changes of infarction occur only in those leads overlying or near the site of infarction.

1. *Inferior infarction* involves the diaphragmatic surface of the heart. It is often caused by occlusion of the right coronary artery or its descending branch. The characteristic electrocardiographic changes of infarction can be seen in the inferior leads II, III, and aVF.

2. *Lateral infarction* involves the left lateral wall of the heart. It is often due to occlusion of the left circumflex artery. Changes will occur in the left lateral leads I, aVL, V5, and V6.

3. *Anterior infarction* involves the anterior surface of the left ventricle and is usually caused by occlusion of the LAD artery. Any of the precordial leads (V1 through V6) may show changes.

4. *Posterior infarction* involves the posterior surface of the heart and is usually caused by occlusion of the right coronary artery. There are no leads overlying the posterior wall. The diagnosis must therefore be made by looking for reciprocal changes in the anterior leads, especially V1.

Actually, it is a very simple matter to put electrodes on a patient's back to get a good look at the posterior electrical forces. When this is done (and, unfortunately, it is done only rarely), the ability of the EKG to diagnose a myocardial infarction is greatly enhanced. These so-called 15-lead EKGs, which include two V leads placed on the back (V8 and V9) and one on the right anterior chest wall (V4R), can often detect ST segment elevation in patients with suspected infarction in whom the 12-lead EKG is normal.

Note: Coronary anatomy can vary markedly among individuals, and the precise vessel involved may not always be what one would predict from the EKG.

Inferior Infarcts

Inferior infarction typically results from occlusion of the right coronary artery or its descending branch. Changes occur in leads II, III, and aVF. Reciprocal changes may be seen in the anterior and left lateral leads.

Although in most infarctions, significant Q waves persist for the lifetime of the patient, this is not necessarily true with inferior infarcts. Within half a year, as many as 50% of these patients will lose their criteria for significant Q waves. The presence of small Q waves inferiorly may therefore suggest an old inferior infarction. Remember, however, that small inferior Q waves also may be seen in normal hearts. The clinical history of the patient must be your guide.

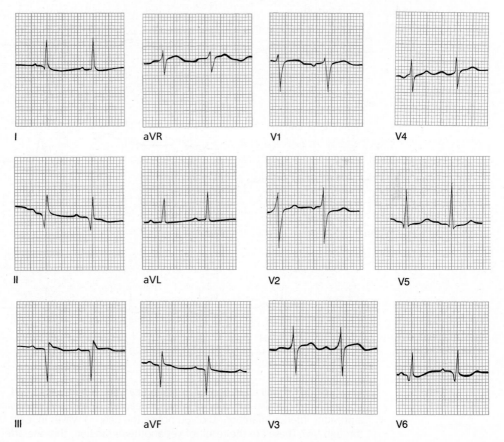

A fully evolved inferior infarction. Deep Q waves can be seen in leads II, III, and aVF.

Lateral Infarction

Lateral infarction may result from occlusion of the left circumflex artery. Changes may be seen in leads I, aVL, V5, and V6. Reciprocal changes may be seen in the inferior leads.

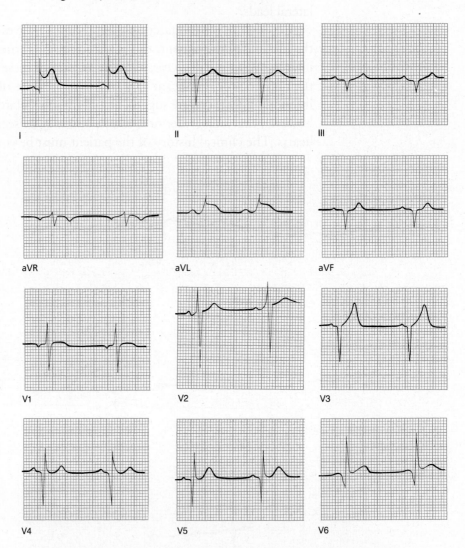

An acute lateral wall infarction. ST elevation can be seen in leads I, aVL, V5, and V6. Note also the deep Q waves in leads II, III, and aVF, signifying a previous inferior infarction. Did you notice the deep Q waves in leads V3 through V6? These are the result of yet another infarction, this one affecting another portion of the left ventricle, that occurred years ago.

Anterior Infarcts

Anterior infarction may result from occlusion of the LAD. Changes are seen in the precordial leads (V1 through V6). If the left main artery is occluded, an anterolateral infarction may result, with changes in the precordial leads and in leads I and aVL. Reciprocal changes are seen inferiorly.

The loss of anterior electrical forces in anterior infarction is not always associated with Q wave formation. In some patients, there may be only a loss or diminishment of the normal pattern of precordial R wave progression. As you already know, under normal circumstances, the precordial leads show a progressive increase in the height of each successive R wave as one moves from V1 to V5. In normal hearts, the amplitude of the R waves should increase at least 1 mV per lead as you progress from V1 to V4 (and often V5). This pattern may vanish with anterior infarction, and the result is called *poor R wave progression*. Even in the absence of significant Q waves, poor R wave progression may signify an anterior infarction.

Poor R wave progression is not specific for the diagnosis of anterior infarction. It also can be seen with right ventricular hypertrophy, in patients with chronic lung disease, and—perhaps most often—with improper lead placement.

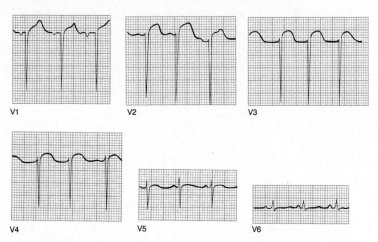

An anterior infarction with poor R wave progression across the precordium.

Posterior Infarction

Posterior infarction typically results from an occlusion of the right coronary artery. Because none of the conventional leads overlie the posterior wall, the diagnosis requires finding reciprocal changes in the anterior leads. In other words, because we can't look for ST segment elevation and Q waves in nonexistent posterior leads, we have to look for *ST segment depression* and *tall R waves* in the anterior leads, notably lead V1. Posterior infarctions are the mirror images of anterior infarctions on the EKG.

The normal QRS complex in lead V1 consists of a small R wave and a deep S wave; therefore, the presence of a tall R wave, particularly with accompanying ST segment depression, should be easy to spot. In the appropriate clinical setting, the presence of an R wave of greater amplitude than the corresponding S wave is highly suggestive of a posterior infarction.

Another helpful clue comes from the blood supply of the heart. Because the inferior wall usually has the same blood supply as the posterior wall, there will often be evidence of accompanying infarction of the inferior wall.

One caveat: you will recall that the presence of a large R wave exceeding the amplitude of the accompanying S wave in lead V1 is also one criterion for the diagnosis of right ventricular hypertrophy. The diagnosis of right ventricular hypertrophy, however, also requires the presence of right axis deviation, which is not present in posterior infarction.

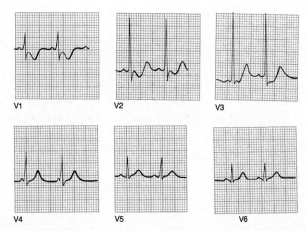

A posterior infarction. In lead V1, the R wave is larger than the S wave. There is also ST depression and T wave inversion in leads V1 and V2.

Where is the infarct? Is it acute?

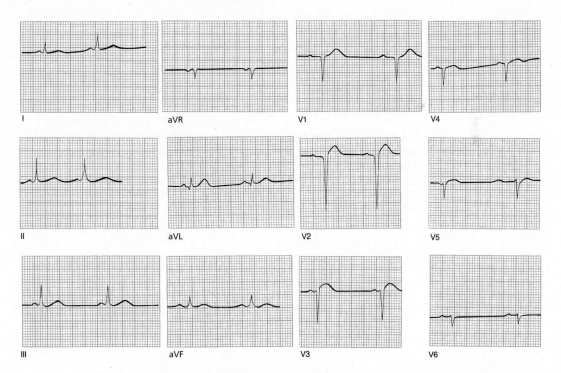

This is an example of an evolving anterior infarction. There is ST segment elevation in leads V2 and V3 as well as poor R wave progression.

Where is the infarct? Is it acute?

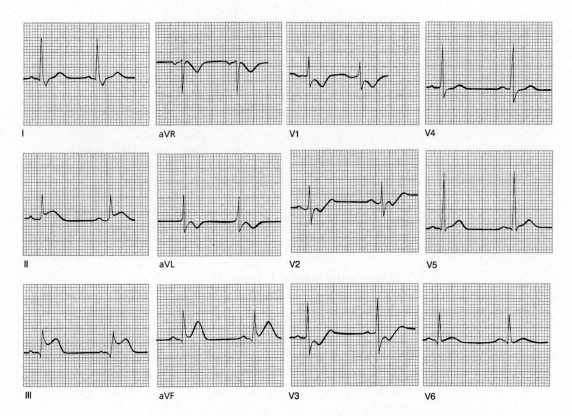

I aVR V1 V4

II aVL V2 V5

III aVF V3 V6

This tracing shows an acute posterior and inferior infarction (remember how we said that most posterior infarctions are accompanied by evidence of inferior infarction?). ST segment elevation with peaked T waves can be seen in leads II, III, and aVF, indicating an acute inferior infarction. There is also evidence of posterior wall involvement, with a tall R wave, ST segment depression, and T wave inversion in lead V1.

Non–Q Wave Myocardial Infarctions

Not all myocardial infarctions produce Q waves. It was previously thought that the production of Q waves required infarction of the entire thickness of the myocardial wall, whereas an absence of Q waves indicated infarction of only a portion of the inner layer of the myocardial wall called the subendocardium. Cardiologists therefore spoke of infarctions as being transmural or subendocardial.

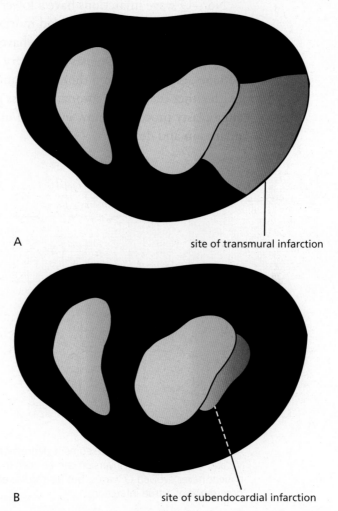

A   site of transmural infarction

B   site of subendocardial infarction

Slices of the heart as seen from above with the large cavity on the right representing the left ventricle. Depiction of (*A*) a transmural infarction and (*B*) a subendocardial infarction.

However, pathologic studies have found little consistent correlation between the evolution of Q waves and whether an infarction is transmural or subendocardial. Some transmural infarctions fail to produce Q waves, and some subendocardial infarctions do produce Q waves. For this reason, the old terminology, however descriptive, has been dropped and replaced by the far less picturesque terms "Q wave infarctions" and "non–Q wave infarctions."

The only EKG changes seen with non–Q wave infarctions are T wave inversion and ST segment depression.

Non–Q wave infarctions have a lower initial mortality rate and a higher risk for later infarction and mortality than Q wave infarctions. Non–Q wave infarctions seem to behave like small, incomplete infarctions, and cardiologists take a very aggressive stance with these patients, evaluating them thoroughly and intervening therapeutically (with either traditional coronary bypass grafting or any of the various angioplasty procedures now in vogue) in an effort to prevent further infarction and death.

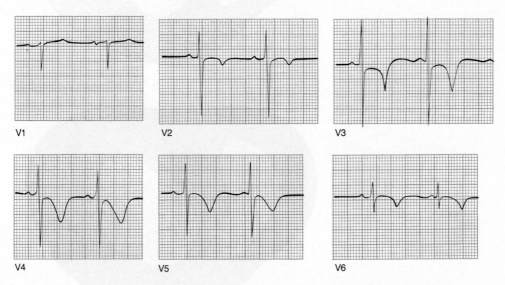

A non–Q wave infarction. ST segment depression is most prominent in leads V2 and V3, and T wave inversion can be seen in leads V2 through V6. This patient never evolved Q waves, but his cardiac enzymes soared, confirming occurrence of a true infarction.

A condition that can closely mimic an acute myocardial infarction on the EKG, complete with T wave inversions and ST segment elevations, is termed **Apical Ballooning Syndrome.** As many as 2% of patients, mostly elderly women, who have what appears to be an acute infarction on EKG will prove to have this syndrome instead. The EKG changes reflect a ballooning of the left ventricle, often brought on by stress (typically emotional stress, hence the syndrome has sometimes been called *broken heart syndrome*), but the precise cause is not well understood. One of the leading theories posits a state of excessive catecholamine stimulation. Troponin levels can be elevated, although rarely as high as in an acute infarction, and there is no evidence of underlying coronary artery disease should the patient be brought to the catheterization lab. As many as 50% of these patients may develop transient heart failure and even go into shock. Patients generally improve over several weeks.

Angina

Angina is the typical chest pain associated with coronary artery disease. A patient with angina may ultimately go on to experience an infarction or may remain stable for many years. An EKG taken during an anginal attack will show *ST segment depression* or *T wave inversion*.

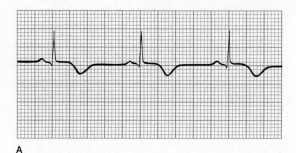

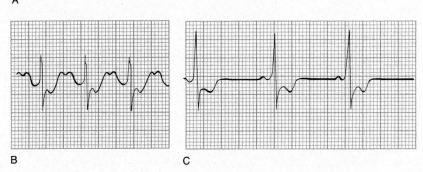

Three examples of the EKG changes that can accompany angina: (*A*) T wave inversion; (*B*) ST segment depression; and (*C*) ST segment depression with T wave inversion (the ST segment and T waves merge seamlessly).

The two ways to distinguish the ST segment depression of angina from that of non–Q wave infarctions are the clinical picture and the time course. With angina, the ST segments usually return to baseline shortly after the attack has subsided. With a non–Q wave infarction, the ST segments remain down for at least 48 hours. Cardiac enzyme levels will be elevated with infarction but not with uncomplicated angina.

Prinzmetal's Angina

There is one type of angina that is associated with ST segment *elevation*. Whereas typical angina is usually brought on by exertion and is the result of progressive atherosclerotic cardiovascular disease, Prinzmetal's angina can occur at any time and, in many patients, results from coronary artery spasm. Presumably, the ST segment elevation reflects reversible transmural injury. The contours of the ST segments often will not have the rounded, domed appearance of true infarction, and the ST segments will return quickly to baseline when the patient is given antianginal medication (*e.g.*, nitroglycerin).

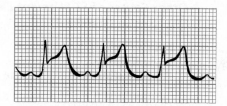

Prinzmetal's angina, with ST segment elevation.

Patients with Prinzmetal's angina actually fall into two groups: those with no atherosclerotic disease whose pain is due solely to coronary artery spasm and those with some underlying atherosclerotic disease who may or may not have superimposed spasm. The EKG does not help to distinguish between these two groups.

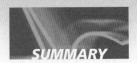

SUMMARY   The ST Segment in Ischemic Cardiac Disease

ST Segment Elevation

May be seen with an evolving transmural infarction or with Prinzmetal's angina

ST Segment Depression

May be seen with typical angina or with a non–Q wave infarction

Other Causes of ST Segment Elevation (many of these will be discussed in Chapter 7)

    J point elevation

    Apical ballooning syndrome

    Acute pericarditis

    Acute myocarditis

    Hyperkalemia

    Pulmonary embolism

    Brugada syndrome

    Hypothermia

The status of the ST segment in patients who present with acute ischemic pain is the major determinant of what kind of therapy they should receive. Patients who present with acute ST segment elevation on their EKG need immediate reperfusion therapy, either thrombolysis or angioplasty. Those with ST segment depression or no ST segment changes can usually be managed more conservatively. However, patients in this latter group should receive aggressive evaluation and therapy if they are at high risk for infarction (*e.g.*, if their cardiac enzymes are elevated, or if they have had a prior angioplasty or bypass grafting).

Limitations of the EKG in Diagnosing an Infarction

Because the electrocardiographic picture of an evolving myocardial infarction typically includes T wave changes, ST segment changes, and Q wave formation, any underlying cardiac condition that masks these effects by distorting the T wave, ST segment, and QRS complex will render electrocardiographic diagnosis of an infarction extremely difficult. Such conditions that we have already discussed are Wolff-Parkinson-White (WPW) syndrome, left ventricular hypertrophy, and left bundle branch block. Right bundle branch block is of less concern because almost all infarctions involve the left ventricle.

Various criteria and algorithms have been devised and tested to aid in the EKG assessment of myocardial infarction in patients with left bundle branch block. None are perfect, as they lack sufficient sensitivity to be uniformly reliable. However, in the setting of left bundle branch block, the presence of ST segment elevation of at least 1 mm in any lead with a predominant R wave is strongly suggestive of an evolving infarction.

In patients with WPW syndrome, the delta waves are often negative in the inferior leads (II, III, and aVF). This pattern is therefore often referred to as a *pseudoinfarct pattern* because the delta waves may resemble Q waves. The short PR interval is the one remaining clue that, in this instance, can distinguish WPW from an infarction on the EKG.

Stress Testing

Stress testing, also called exercise tolerance testing, is a noninvasive method of assessing the presence and severity of coronary artery disease. It is by no means flawless (false-positive and false-negative results abound), but it is still the best noninvasive screening procedure available. The alternative—taking all candidates directly to cardiac catheterization—is neither feasible nor desirable. Other tests that are being added to the investigatory armamentarium and that are proving helpful include *rapid CT scanning* of the heart, which provides a measure of the degree of atherosclerosis in the coronary arteries but does not reliably predict the degree of blockage at any one specific site, and *CT angiography*, which may provide a useful intermediary step between stress testing and catheterization but which carries all the risks associated with a high dye load.

Stress testing is usually done by having the patient ambulate on a treadmill, although stationary bicycles have been used just as effectively. The patient is hooked up to an EKG monitor, and a rhythm strip is monitored throughout the test. A complete 12-lead EKG is usually taken every minute and at the peak of exercise. Every few minutes, the speed and angle of incline of the treadmill are increased until (1) the patient cannot continue for any reason; (2) the patient's maximal heart rate is achieved; (3) symptoms supervene; or (4) significant changes are seen on the EKG.

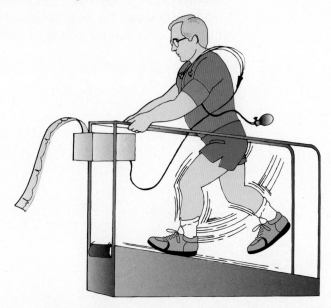

The physiology behind stress testing is simple. The graded exercise protocol causes a safe and gradual increase in the patient's heart rate and systolic blood pressure. The product of the patient's blood pressure multiplied by his heart rate, called the *double product*, is a good measure of myocardial oxygen consumption. If cardiac oxygen demands exceed consumption, electrocardiographic changes and sometimes symptoms of myocardial ischemia may occur.

Significant coronary artery disease of one or several coronary arteries limits blood flow to the myocardium and hence limits oxygen consumption. Although a patient's resting EKG may be normal, the increased demands of exercise may bring out evidence of subclinical coronary artery disease.

With a positive test for coronary artery disease, the EKG will reveal *ST segment depression.* T wave changes are too nonspecific to have any meaning in this setting.

There is a wealth of literature questioning precisely what constitutes significant ST segment depression during an exercise test. It is generally acknowledged that ST segment depression of greater than 1 mm that is horizontal or downsloping and persists for more than 0.08 seconds is suggestive of coronary artery disease. If a depression of 2 mm is used as the criterion, the number of false-positive results is greatly reduced, but the number of false-negative results increases. Occasionally, upsloping ST segments may signify coronary artery disease, but the number of false-positive results is very high.

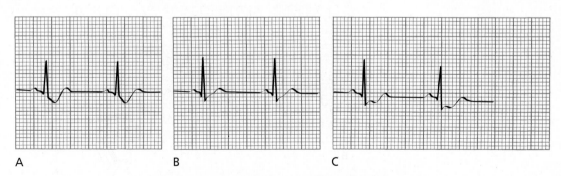

A   B   C

(*A*) Downsloping ST depression. (*B*) Upsloping ST depression. (*C*) Horizontal ST depression. Only *A* and *C* are highly suggestive of coronary artery disease.

The earlier in the test that ST segment depression occurs—particularly if the changes persist several minutes into the recovery period—the greater the likelihood that coronary artery disease is present and the greater the possibility that the left main coronary artery or several coronary arteries are involved. The onset of symptoms and falling blood pressure are particularly important signs, and the test must be stopped immediately.

The incidence of false-positive and false-negative results is dependent on the patient population that is being tested. A positive test in a young, healthy individual with no symptoms and no risk factors for coronary artery disease is likely to be a false test. On the other hand, a positive test in an elderly man with chest pain, a prior infarction, and hypertension is much more likely to be a true-positive result. In no one does a negative test result absolutely exclude the possibility of coronary artery disease.

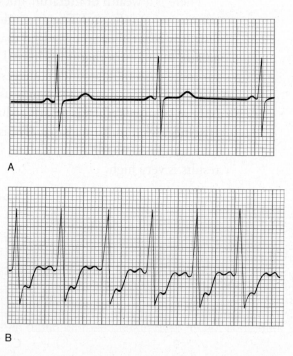

A

B

(A) A patient's resting EKG. (B) The same lead in the same patient 12 minutes into an exercise test. Note the prominent ST segment depression associated with the increased heart rate.

Indications for stress testing include the following:

1. The differential diagnosis of chest pain in someone whose baseline EKG is normal

2. The evaluation of a patient who has recently had an infarction, in order to assess his or her prognosis and need for further invasive testing, such as cardiac catheterization

3. The evaluation of individuals over 40 years of age who have risk factors for coronary artery disease, particularly diabetes mellitus, peripheral vascular disease, a history of a prior myocardial infarction, or a family history of premature heart disease

4. Suspicion of silent ischemia, such as in patients without chest pain but who may complain of shortness of breath, fatigue, palpitations, or erectile dysfunction

5. Stress testing is also frequently done in patients over 40 years of age who want to start an exercise program.

Contraindications include any acute systemic illness, severe aortic stenosis, uncontrolled congestive heart failure, severe hypertension, angina at rest, and the presence of a significant arrhythmia.

Mortality from the procedure is very low, but resuscitation equipment should always be available.

Both the sensitivity and specificity of the exercise stress test can be increased by (1) doing an **echocardiogram** before and after the procedure, looking for exercise-induced changes in wall motion that might signify myocardium in jeopardy, or (2) injecting the patient with **radioactive imaging agents** during the test and then recording images of the heart. The myocardium extracts the radiotracer from the coronary circulation, but regions of compromised blood flow will be unable to extract the radiotracer. Therefore, in a normal test, myocardial scintigraphy will reveal uniform uptake of the isotope by the left ventricle, but in a patient with coronary stenosis, a large perfusion defect may be seen. Some time later, a second film is taken, at which point the heart is no longer under stress. The perfusion defect may now disappear, indicating that the stenosed coronary artery is supplying blood to viable myocardium; medical or surgical intervention to treat the stenosis may therefore preserve the affected region of the left ventricle. On the other hand, if the perfusion defect does not disappear on the second film, one can conclude that the region in question is no longer metabolically capable of taking up the tracer and is therefore most likely infarcted; restoring blood flow to that region of the heart is unlikely to be of any benefit.

In patients who are unable to exercise, there are alternatives to the traditional stress test. These include **adenosine stress testing** and **dobutamine stress testing.**

Adenosine, given intravenously, produces transient coronary vasodilatation, increasing coronary blood flow up to 400%. Vessels with significant stenosis are unable to vasodilate as effectively as healthy vessels, and the territory of the heart they supply will thus show less uptake of the radioactive tracer. Typically, there are no diagnostic EKG changes during this test.

A dobutamine stress test mimics the stress of exercise on the heart. Dobutamine is an adrenaline-like agent that is given in incremental doses over several minutes. In patients with coronary artery disease, EKG changes just like those induced by exercise may be seen, and transient wall motion abnormalities will be seen on an accompanying echocardiogram.

9.

Joan L. is a 62-year-old business executive. She is on an important business trip and spends the night at a hotel downtown. Early the next morning, she is awakened with shortness of breath and severe chest pressure that radiates into her jaw and left arm. She gets out of bed and takes Pepto-Bismol, but the pain does not go away. Feeling dizzy and nauseated, she sits down and phones the front desk. Her symptoms are relayed by phone to the doctor covering the hotel, who immediately orders an ambulance to take her to the local emergency room. She arrives there only 2 hours after the onset of her symptoms, which have continued unabated despite three sublingual nitroglycerin tablets given to her during the ambulance ride.

In the emergency room, a 12-lead EKG reveals the following:

Is she having an infarction? If so, can you tell if it is acute and what region of the heart is affected?

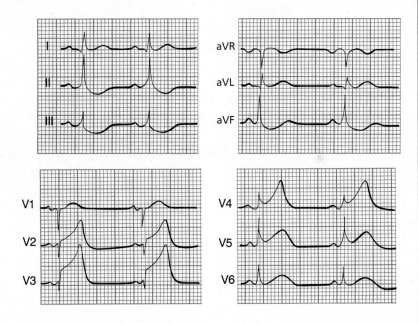

The EKG shows ST segment elevation in leads V2 through V5. There are no Q waves. Joan is in the throes of an acute anterior myocardial infarction.

Joan's prompt arrival in the emergency room, the elevated ST segments, and the absence of Q waves on the EKG mean that she is an excellent candidate for either thrombolytic therapy or acute coronary angioplasty. Unfortunately, she relates that only 1 month ago she suffered a mild hemorrhagic stroke, leaving her with some weakness in her left arm and leg, and making the risks of thrombolytic therapy prohibitive. In addition, acute angioplasty is not available at this small community hospital, and the nearest large medical center is several hours away. Therefore, doing the best they can under the circumstances, the medical staff have Joan admitted to the cardiac care unit (CCU) to be monitored. Her pain is controlled with morphine and intravenous nitroglycerin, and she is given intravenous beta-blockers to reduce sympathetic nervous system stimulation of her heart. Aspirin is also given, but all other anticoagulant agents are withheld because of her stroke history. Her first troponin level comes back elevated.

Late on the first night of her hospital stay, one of the nurses notices peculiar beats on her EKG:

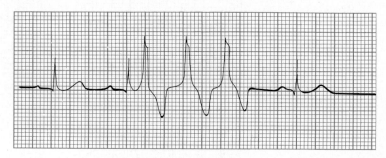

What are they?

The patient's normal sinus rhythm is being interrupted by a run of three consecutive premature ventricular contractions (PVCs). In the setting of an acute infarction, antiarrhythmic therapy is often given immediately because these PVCs can trigger ventricular tachycardia and fibrillation.

The next morning, Joan's EKG looks like this. What has changed?

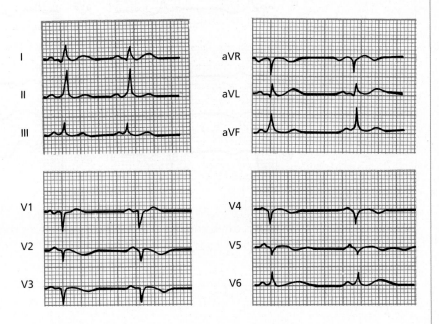

Joan's EKG shows that all ventricular ectopy has been suppressed. It also shows new Q waves in the anterior leads, consistent with full evolution of an anterior infarct.

Later in the afternoon, Joan again begins to experience chest pain. A repeat EKG is taken. What has changed?

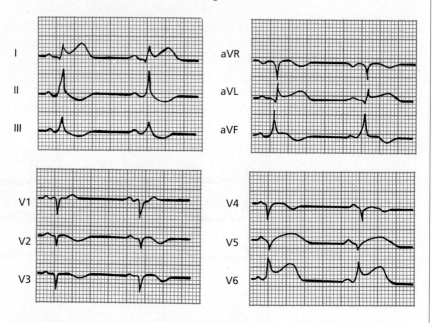

Joan is extending her infarct. New ST elevations can be seen in the left lateral leads.

A few hours later, she complains of light-headedness, and another EKG is performed. Now what do you see?

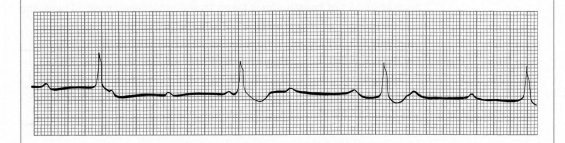

Joan has gone into third-degree AV block. Serious conduction blocks are most commonly seen in anterior infarctions. Her light-headedness is due to inadequate cardiac output in the face of a ventricular escape rhythm of approximately 35 beats per minute. Pacemaker insertion is mandatory.

A pacemaker is placed without difficulty, and Joan suffers no further complications during her hospital stay. One week later, ambulatory and pain free, she is discharged. The morning after returning home, she again awakens short of breath and is taken to the emergency room. There, she is found to be in congestive heart failure. A cardiac echogram reveals markedly diminished left ventricular function as a result of her large myocardial infarction. She is treated in the hospital and is discharged 3 days later on a diuretic, a beta-blocker and an angiotensin-converting enzyme (ACE) inhibitor. No further problems develop, and she is able to return to her normal life at home and at work.

This case is very typical of the sort of thing you see over and over again in hospitals across the country. It emphasizes how critical the EKG is in diagnosing and managing patients with acute myocardial infarctions. With Joan, an EKG confirmed the initial suspicion that she was having an infarct. In the CCU, electrocardiographic surveillance permitted the diagnosis of further infarction and accompanying rhythm and conduction disturbances and guided major therapeutic decisions.

7. Finishing Touches

In this chapter you will learn:

1 | that the EKG can be changed by a whole variety of other cardiac and noncardiac disorders. We will discuss the most important of these as well as several other critical areas where the role of the EKG is paramount:

A electrolyte disturbances

B hypothermia

C digitalis effects, both therapeutic and toxic

D medications that prolong the QT interval

E other cardiac disorders (*e.g.,* pericarditis, cardiomyopathy, and myocarditis)

F pulmonary disorders

G central nervous system disease

H sudden cardiac death in persons without coronary artery disease

I the athlete's heart

2 | about the cases of Amos T., whose EKG proves to be the key to unraveling an emergent, life-threatening noncardiac condition and that of Ursula U., almost done in by some very common medications.

There are a number of medications, electrolyte disturbances, and other disorders that can substantially alter the normal pattern of the EKG. It is not always clear *why* the EKG is so sensitive to such a seemingly diffuse array of conditions, but it is, and you've got to know about them.

In some of these instances, the EKG may actually be the most sensitive indicator of impending catastrophe. In others, subtle electrocardiographic changes may be an early clue to a previously unsuspected problem. In still others, the electrocardiographic alteration may be incidental, vaguely interesting, and hardly illuminating.

Electrolyte Disturbances

Alterations in the serum levels of potassium and calcium can profoundly alter the EKG.

Hyperkalemia

Hyperkalemia produces a progressive evolution of changes in the EKG that can culminate in ventricular fibrillation and death. *The presence of electrocardiographic changes is a better measure of clinically significant potassium toxicity than the serum potassium level.*

As the potassium begins to rise, the T waves across the entire 12-lead EKG begin to peak. This effect can easily be confused with the peaked T waves of an acute myocardial infarction. One difference is that the changes in an infarction are confined to those leads overlying the area of the infarct, whereas in hyperkalemia, the changes are diffuse.

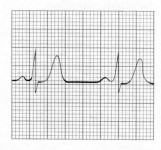

The peaked T waves of hyperkalemia.

With a further increase in the serum potassium, the PR interval becomes prolonged, and the P wave gradually flattens and then disappears.

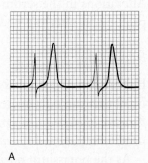

A

As the potassium level rises, P waves are no longer visible. The T waves are even more peaked.

Ultimately, the QRS complex widens until it merges with the T wave, forming a sine wave pattern. Ventricular fibrillation may eventually develop.

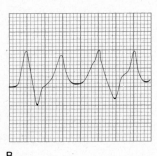

B

Progressive hyperkalemia leads to the classic sine wave pattern. The widened QRS complexes and peaked T waves are almost indistinguishable.

It is important to note that, whereas these changes frequently do occur in the order described as the serum potassium rises, they do not *always* do so. Progression to ventricular fibrillation can occur with devastating suddenness. **Any change in the EKG due to hyperkalemia mandates immediate clinical attention!**

Hypokalemia

With hypokalemia, the EKG may again be a better measure of serious toxicity than the serum potassium level. Three changes can be seen, occurring in no particular order:

- ST segment depression
- Flattening of the T wave
- Appearance of a U wave.

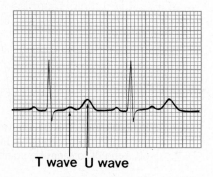

T wave U wave

Hypokalemia. The U waves are even more prominent than the T waves.

The term *U wave* is given to a wave appearing after the T wave in the cardiac cycle. It usually has the same axis as the T wave, and is often best seen in the anterior leads. Its precise physiologic meaning is not fully understood. Although U waves are the most characteristic feature of hypokalemia, they are not in and of themselves diagnostic. Other conditions can produce prominent U waves (central nervous system disease and certain antiarrhythmic drugs, for example) and U waves can sometimes be seen in patients with normal hearts and normal serum potassium levels.

Calcium Disorders

Alterations in the serum calcium primarily affect the QT interval. Hypocalcemia prolongs it; hypercalcemia shortens it. Do you remember a potentially lethal arrhythmia associated with a prolonged QT interval?

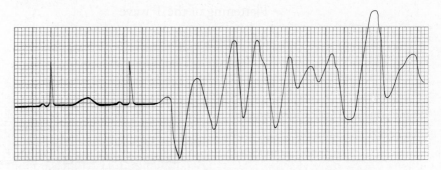

Hypocalcemia. The QT interval is slightly prolonged. A premature ventricular contraction (PVC) falls on the prolonged T wave and sets off a run of torsades de pointes.

Torsades de pointes, a variant of ventricular tachycardia, is seen in patients with prolonged QT intervals.

Hypothermia

As the body temperature dips below 30°C, several changes occur on the EKG:

1. Everything slows down. Sinus bradycardia is common, and all the segments and intervals—PR, QRS, QT, *etc.*—may become prolonged.

2. A distinctive and virtually diagnostic type of ST segment elevation may be seen. It consists of an abrupt ascent right at the J point and then an equally sudden plunge back to baseline. The resultant configuration is called a *J wave* or *Osborn wave*.

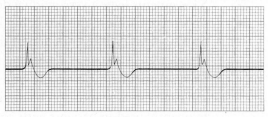

A

Hypothermia. The Osborn waves are very prominent.

3. Various arrhythmias may ultimately supervene. Slow atrial fibrillation is most common, although almost any rhythm disturbance can occur.

4. A muscle tremor artifact due to shivering may complicate the tracing. A similar artifact may be seen in patients with Parkinson's disease. Do not confuse this with atrial flutter.

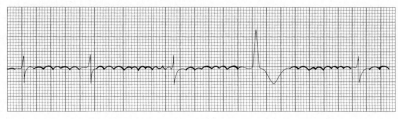

B

A muscle tremor artifact resembles atrial flutter.

Drugs

Digitalis

There are two distinct categories of electrocardiographic alterations caused by digitalis: those associated with *therapeutic* blood levels of the drug and those seen with *toxic* blood levels.

EKG Changes Associated With Therapeutic Blood Levels

Therapeutic levels of digitalis produce characteristic ST segment and T wave changes in most individuals taking the drug. These changes are known as the *digitalis effect* and consist of ST segment depression with flattening or inversion of the T wave. The depressed ST segments have a very gradual downslope, emerging almost imperceptibly from the preceding R wave. This distinctive appearance usually permits differentiation of the digitalis effect from the more symmetric ST segment depression of ischemia; differentiation from ventricular hypertrophy with repolarization abnormalities can sometimes be more problematic, especially because digitalis is frequently used in patients with congestive heart failure who often have left ventricular hypertrophy.

The digitalis effect usually is most prominent in leads with tall R waves. *Remember:* the digitalis effect is normal and predictable and does not necessitate discontinuing the drug.

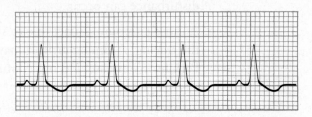

The digitalis effect, with asymmetric ST segment depression.

EKG Changes Associated With Toxic Blood Levels

The *toxic manifestations* of digitalis, on the other hand, may require clinical intervention. Digitalis intoxication can elicit conduction blocks and tachyarrhythmias, alone or in combination.

Sinus Node Suppression

Even at therapeutic blood levels of digitalis, the sinus node can be slowed, particularly in patients with the sick sinus syndrome. At toxic blood levels, sinus exit block or complete sinus node suppression can occur.

Conduction Blocks

Digitalis slows conduction through the AV node and can therefore cause first-, second-, and even third-degree AV block.

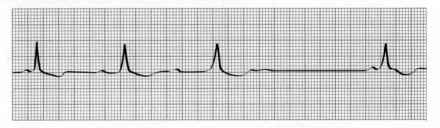

Wenckebach block caused by digitalis intoxication.

The ability of digitalis to slow AV conduction has made it useful in the treatment of supraventricular tachycardias. For example, digitalis can slow the ventricular rate in patients with atrial fibrillation; however, the ability of digitalis to slow the heart rate, best seen when the patients are sitting or lying quietly for their EKG recording, is commonly lost during exertion. Beta-blockers, such as atenolol or metoprolol, have a similar effect on AV conduction and may control the rate better when there is increased adrenergic tone (*e.g.*, during exercise or stress).

Tachyarrhythmias

Because digitalis enhances the automatic behavior of all cardiac conducting cells, causing them to act more like pacemakers, there is no tachyarrhythmia that digitalis cannot cause. Paroxysmal atrial tachycardia (PAT) and PVCs are the most common, junctional rhythms are fairly common, and atrial flutter and fibrillation are the least common.

Combinations

The combination of PAT with second-degree AV block is the most characteristic rhythm disturbance of digitalis intoxication. The conduction block is usually 2:1 but may vary unpredictably. Digitalis is the most common, but not the only, cause of PAT with block.

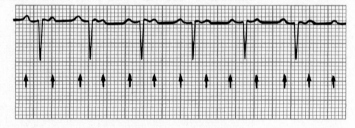

Paroxysmal atrial tachycardia (PAT) with 2:1 block. The *arrows* point to each P wave.

Medications That Prolong the QT Interval

Among the medications that can increase the QT interval are the antiarrhythmic agents (*e.g.*, sotalol, quinidine, procainamide, disopyramide, amiodarone, dofetilide, and dronedarone). These agents are used to treat arrhythmias, but by increasing the QT interval they can paradoxically increase the risk for serious ventricular tachyarrhythmias. The QT interval must be carefully monitored in all patients taking these medications, and the drug should be stopped if substantial—usually more than 25%—prolongation occurs.

Other medications that can prolong the QT interval include the tricyclic antidepressants, the phenothiazines, erythromycin, the quinolone antibiotics, and various antifungal medications.

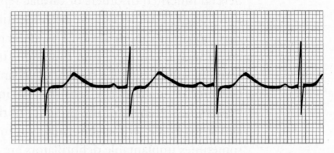

The prolonged QT interval on this tracing mandated reducing the patient's sotalol dosage.

More on the QT Interval

Several inherited disorders of cardiac repolarization associated with long QT intervals have been identified and linked to specific chromosomal abnormalities. The cause in almost half of genotyped individuals is one of various mutations in a gene that encodes pore-forming subunits of the membrane channels that generate a slow K^+ current that is adrenergic sensitive. All individuals in these families need to be screened for the presence of the genetic defect with resting and stress EKGs. If the abnormality is found, beta-blocking drugs and sometimes implantable defibrillators are recommended because the risk for sudden death from a lethal arrhythmia is greatly increased, especially when the patient is in childhood or early adulthood. These patients must also be restricted from competitive sports (although modest exercise without "adrenalin bursts" can be encouraged and guided by the results of the exercise stress test) and must never take any drugs that can prolong the QT interval. In a few patients who are particularly susceptible to the adverse effects of increased adrenergic tone, left cervical–thoracic sympathetic denervation may be needed.

How to Measure the QT Interval Accurately

Because the QT interval varies normally with the heart rate, a *corrected QT interval,* or QTc, is used to assess absolute QT prolongation. The QTc adjusts for differences in the heart rate by dividing the QT interval by the square root of the R-R interval—that is, the square root of one cardiac cycle:

$$QTc = \frac{QT}{\sqrt{RR}}$$

The QTc should not exceed 500 ms during therapy with any medication that can prolong the QT interval (550 ms if there is an underlying bundle branch block); adhering to this rule will reduce the risk for ventricular arrhythmias. The formula for determining the QTc is most accurate at heart rates between 50 and 120 beats per minute; at the extremes of heart rate, its usefulness is limited.

Other Cardiac Disorders

Pericarditis

Acute pericarditis may cause ST segment elevation and T wave flattening or inversion. These changes can easily be confused with an evolving infarction, as can the clinical picture. Certain features of the EKG can be helpful in differentiating pericarditis from infarction:

1. The ST segment and T wave changes in pericarditis tend to be diffuse (although not always), involving far more leads than the localized effect of infarction.

2. In pericarditis, T wave inversion usually occurs only after the ST segments have returned to baseline. In infarction, T wave inversion usually precedes normalization of the ST segments.

3. In pericarditis, Q wave formation does not occur.

4. The PR interval is sometimes depressed.

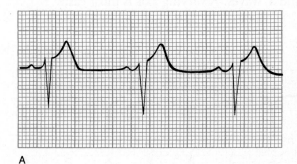

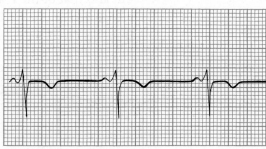

A   B

(*A*) Lead V3 shows the ST segment elevation of acute pericarditis. (*B*) The same lead several days later shows that the ST segments have returned to baseline and the T waves have inverted. There are no Q waves.

Formation of a substantial *pericardial effusion* dampens the electrical output of the heart, resulting in low voltage in all leads. The ST segment and T wave changes of pericarditis may still be evident.

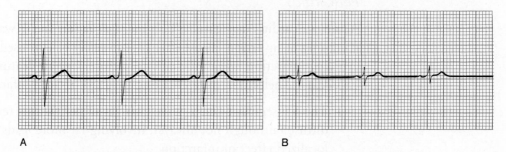

A   B

Lead I before (*A*) and after (*B*) the development of a pericardial effusion. Decreased voltage is the only significant change.

If an effusion is sufficiently large, the heart may actually rotate freely within the fluid-filled sac. This produces the phenomenon of *electrical alternans* in which the electrical axis of the heart varies with each beat. This can affect not only the axis of the QRS complex but also that of the P and T waves. A varying axis is most easily recognized on the EKG by the varying amplitude of each waveform from beat to beat.

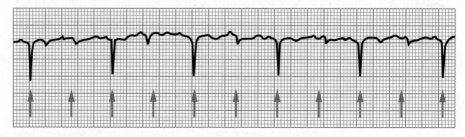

Electrical alternans. The *arrows* point to each QRS complex.

Hypertrophic Obstructive Cardiomyopathy

We have already discussed hypertrophic obstructive cardiomyopathy (HOCM), also known as idiopathic hypertrophic subaortic stenosis, in the case of Tom L. Many patients with HOCM have normal EKGs, but left ventricular hypertrophy and left axis deviation are not uncommon. Q waves may sometimes be seen laterally and occasionally inferiorly. These do not represent infarction.

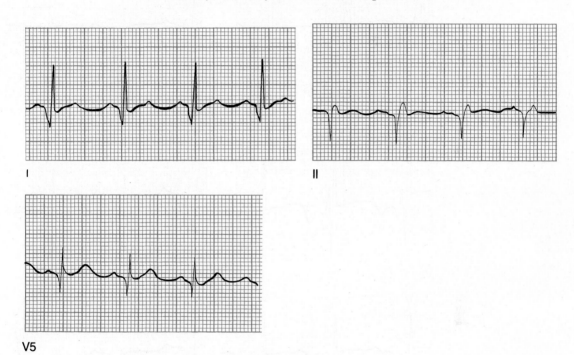

I

II

V5

HOCM. Significant Q waves can be seen in both lateral and inferior leads.

Myocarditis

Any diffuse inflammatory process involving the myocardium can produce a number of changes on the EKG. Most common are conduction blocks, especially bundle branch blocks and hemiblocks.

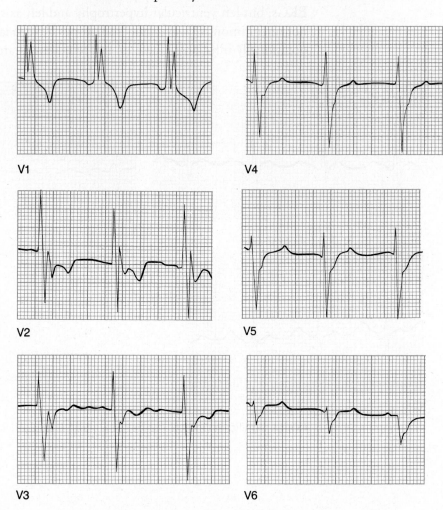

Right bundle branch block in a patient with active myocarditis following a viral infection.

Pulmonary Disorders

Chronic Obstructive Pulmonary Disease (COPD)

The EKG of a patient with long-standing emphysema may show low voltage, right axis deviation, and poor R wave progression in the precordial leads. The low voltage is caused by the dampening effects of the expanded residual volume of air trapped in the lungs. Right axis deviation is caused by the expanded lungs forcing the heart into a vertical or even rightward-oriented position, as well as by the pressure overload hypertrophy from pulmonary hypertension.

COPD can lead to chronic cor pulmonale and right-sided congestive heart failure. The EKG may then show right atrial enlargement (P pulmonale) and right ventricular hypertrophy with repolarization abnormalities.

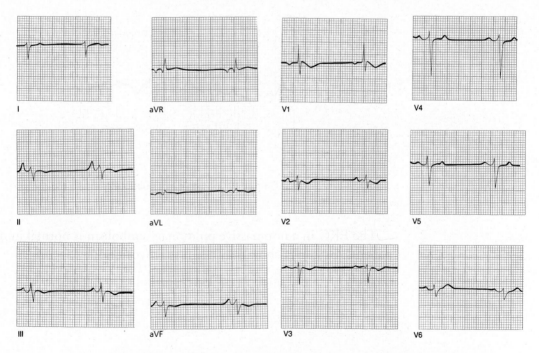

Chronic obstructive pulmonary disease. Note the low voltage, extreme right axis deviation, right atrial enlargement (in lead II), and precordial criteria for right ventricular hypertrophy.

Acute Pulmonary Embolism

A sudden massive pulmonary embolus can profoundly alter the EKG. Findings may include the following:

1. A pattern of right ventricular hypertrophy with repolarization changes, presumably due to acute right ventricular dilatation

2. Right bundle branch block

3. A large S wave in lead I and a deep Q wave in lead III. This is called the *S1Q3 pattern*. The T wave in lead III may also be inverted. Unlike an inferior infarction, in which Q waves are usually seen in at least two of the inferior leads, the Q waves in an acute pulmonary embolus are generally limited to lead III.

4. A number of arrhythmias may be produced; most common are sinus tachycardia and atrial fibrillation.

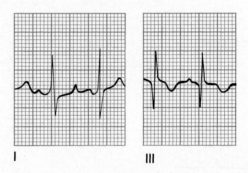

The S1Q3 pattern of a massive pulmonary embolus.

The EKG in a nonmassive pulmonary embolism is normal in most patients, or it may show only a sinus tachycardia.

Central Nervous System Disease

Central nervous system (CNS) catastrophes, such as a subarachnoid bleed or cerebral infarction, can produce diffuse T wave inversion and prominent U waves. The T waves are typically very deep and very wide, and their contour is usually symmetrical (unlike the asymmetrical inverted T waves of secondary repolarization associated with ventricular hypertrophy). Sinus bradycardia also is commonly seen. These changes are believed to be due to involvement of the autonomic nervous system.

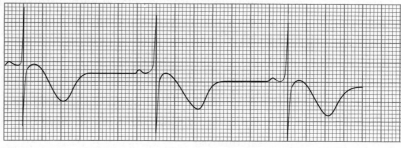

V4

Deeply inverted, wide T waves in lead V4 in a patient with a central nervous system bleed.

Sudden Cardiac Death

By far the most common cause of sudden cardiac death is underlying atherosclerosis (coronary artery disease) triggering infarction and/or arrhythmia. However, there are other causes as well, some of which we have discussed. These include the following:

Hypertrophic cardiomyopathy

Long QT interval syndrome, acquired or congenital

Arrhythmogenic right ventricular dysplasia, a heritable cardiomyopathy associated with fibrofatty infiltration of the right ventricular myocardium, and an important cause of ventricular arrhythmias and sudden death

Wolff-Parkinson-White syndrome

Viral myocarditis

Infiltrative diseases of the myocardium (*e.g.*, amyloidosis and sarcoidosis)

Valvular heart disease

Drug abuse (especially cocaine and amphetamines)

Commotio cordis, in which blunt force to the chest causes ventricular fibrillation

Anomalous origin of the coronary arteries, in which constriction of the artery by surrounding tissue—exacerbating by the increased myocardial contractions of exercise—can cause ventricular fibrillation

Brugada syndrome.

Brugada syndrome occurs in structurally normal hearts, and in this way resembles the long QT syndromes. It is inherited as an autosomal dominant trait, yet it is much more common in men (especially those in their 20s and 30s) than in women. The cause in some patients is a genetic mutation affecting voltage-dependent sodium channels during repolarization. Brugada syndrome can be identified by a specific set of abnormalities on the EKG: a pattern resembling right bundle branch block and ST segment elevation in leads V1, V2, and V3.

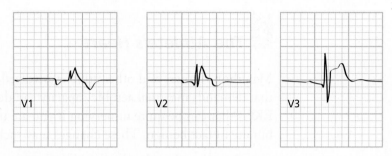

Brugada syndrome. Note the right bundle branch pattern and ST elevation.

The importance of Brugada syndrome lies in its propensity to cause ventricular arrhythmias that can cause sudden death. The most typical of these is a fast polymorphic ventricular tachycardia that looks just like torsades de pointes. Sudden death is most likely to occur during sleep. However, beta-blockers are of no help in this condition. Implantable cardiac defibrillators are a critical component of management. All family members of an affected patient must be screened for this condition.

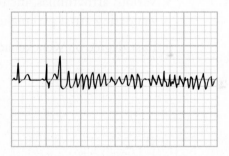

Polymorphous ventricular tachycardia with unusually narrow QRS complexes in a patient with Brugada syndrome.

The Athlete's Heart

Marathon runners and other athletes involved in endurance training that demands maximal aerobic capacity can develop alterations in their EKGs that can be quite unnerving if you are unfamiliar with them, but are in fact benign. These changes may include the following:

1. A resting sinus bradycardia, sometimes even below 30 beats per minute! Rather than a cause for concern, this profound sinus bradycardia is a testimony to the efficiency of their cardiovascular system.

2. Nonspecific ST segment and T wave changes. Typically, these consist of ST segment elevation in the precordial leads with T wave flattening or inversion.

3. Criteria for left ventricular hypertrophy and sometimes right ventricular hypertrophy

4. Incomplete right bundle branch block

5. Various arrhythmias, including junctional rhythms and a wandering atrial pacemaker

6. First-degree or Wenckebach AV block.

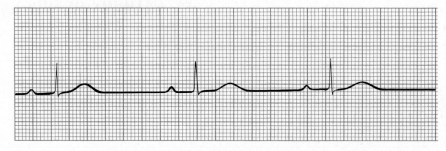

Sinus bradycardia and first-degree AV block in a triathlete.

None of these conditions is cause for concern, nor do they require treatment. More than one endurance athlete, undergoing a routine EKG, has been admitted to the cardiac care unit (CCU) because of unfamiliarity with these changes.

Athletes are at an increased risk of sudden death compared to age-matched populations of nonathletes. The most common causes are disorders of the heart muscle and sudden ventricular arrhythmias. Preparticipation screening in young athletes with a careful physical examination and baseline EKG will prevent some of these deaths, and in certain countries, baseline echocardiograms are obtained as well.

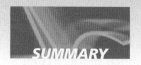

SUMMARY

Miscellaneous Conditions

Electrolyte Disturbances

- *Hyperkalemia:* Evolution of (1) peaked T waves, (2) PR prolongation and P wave flattening, and (3) QRS widening. Ultimately, the QRS complexes and T waves merge to form a sine wave, and ventricular fibrillation may develop.

- *Hypokalemia:* ST depression, T wave flattening, U waves

- *Hypocalcemia:* Prolonged QT interval

- *Hypercalcemia:* Shortened QT interval.

Hypothermia

- Osborn waves, prolonged intervals, sinus bradycardia, slow atrial fibrillation. Beware of muscle tremor artifact.

Drugs

- *Digitalis: Therapeutic levels* are associated with ST segment and T wave changes in leads with tall R waves; *toxic levels* are associated with tachyarrhythmias and conduction blocks; PAT with block is most characteristic.

- *Antiarrhythmic agents (and numerous other drugs, see page 270):* Prolonged QT interval, U waves

Other Cardiac Disorders

- *Pericarditis:* Diffuse ST segment and T wave changes. A large effusion can cause low voltage and electrical alternans.

- *Hypertrophic cardiomyopathy:* Ventricular hypertrophy, left axis deviation, septal Q waves

- *Myocarditis:* Conduction blocks

Pulmonary Disorders

- *COPD:* Low voltage, right axis deviation, poor R wave progression. Chronic cor pulmonale can produce P pulmonale and right ventricular hypertrophy with repolarization abnormalities.

- *Acute pulmonary embolism:* Right ventricular hypertrophy with repolarization abnormalities, right bundle branch block, S1Q3. Sinus tachycardia and atrial fibrillation are the most common arrhythmias.

CNS Disease

- Diffuse T wave inversion, with T waves typically wide and deep; U waves.

The Athlete's Heart

- Sinus bradycardia, nonspecific ST segment and T wave changes, left and right ventricular hypertrophy, incomplete right bundle branch block, first-degree or Wenckebach AV block, occasional supraventricular arrhythmia.

CASE

10.

Amos T., a 25-year-old graduate student, is brought by ambulance to the emergency room, clutching his chest and looking not at all well. Vital signs show a blood pressure of 90/40 mm Hg and an irregular pulse. His rhythm strip looks like this.

Do you recognize the arrhythmia?

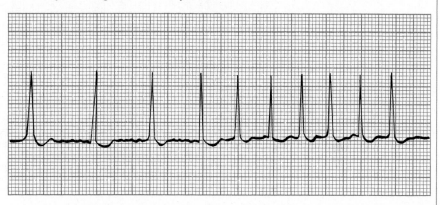

The patient is in atrial fibrillation. There are no P waves, the baseline undulates, and the QRS complexes appear irregularly and are narrow.

Appropriate measures are taken, and Amos is converted back to sinus rhythm, although his rate remains fast at around 100 beats per minute. His blood pressure rises to 130/60 mm Hg. Despite successful conversion of his rhythm, he still complains of severe chest pain and shortness of breath. The emergency room physician wants to treat him immediately for an acute myocardial infarction, but you insist on a good 12-lead EKG first—not an unreasonable request because, except for his tachycardia, his vital signs are stable. The EKG is obtained.

Do you now agree with the emergency room physician's assessment?

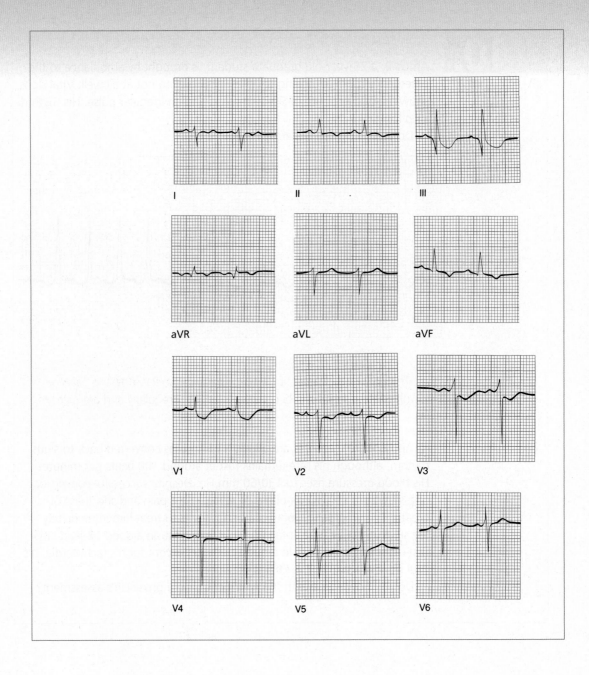

I

II

III

aVR

aVL

aVF

V1

V2

V3

V4

V5

V6

Of course you don't. Hopefully, you noticed some of the following features:

1. The patient now has a rate of 100 beats per minute.

2. A pattern of right ventricular hypertrophy with repolarization abnormalities is present.

3. A deep Q wave is seen in lead III and a deep S wave in lead I, the classic S1Q3 of an acute pulmonary embolus.

Do you now start jumping up and down and scream that the patient has an acute pulmonary embolus? No. You start jumping up and down and scream that the patient *may* have a pulmonary embolus. These EKG findings are suggestive but hardly conclusive. You have done your job well just by raising the issue; appropriate diagnostic steps can now be taken.

Amos is placed on heparin while awaiting his chest CT scan. This is done within the hour, and the diagnosis of a pulmonary embolism is confirmed. Amos remains in the hospital for several days on heparin therapy and is discharged home on oral anticoagulant therapy. There is no recurrence of his pulmonary embolism.

By the way, in case you were wondering why Amos developed a pulmonary embolism, you should know that he had a strong family history of deep venous thrombophlebitis, and a careful hematologic workup found that he had an inherited deficiency of protein S, a normal inhibitor of the coagulation cascade. Now, try to find that in other EKG books!

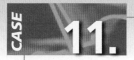

CASE 11.

Ursula U. was recently seen at your local hospital for pyelonephritis (a urinary tract infection involving the kidney) and discharged home on the antibiotic, trimethoprim–sulfamethoxazole. She seeks routine follow-up care with you. She is fairly new in town and new to your practice. Her infection certainly seems to be responding well to the antibiotic, but you note that her blood pressure is a little elevated at 145/95. She tells you that she is currently taking the blood pressure medication, lisinopril, an angiotensin-converting enzyme inhibitor, but has not seen a physician since the drug was prescribed. Something clicks in your head, and you obtain an EKG. Here are the tracings from just her augmented limb leads. What do you see?

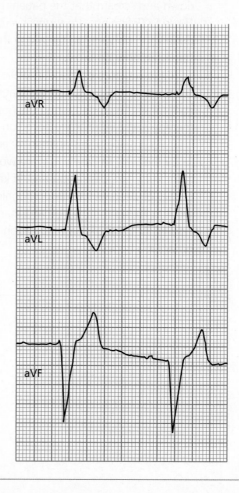

This looks like pretty wild stuff. But analyze this slowly: the QRS complexes are clearly very wide, and there are no visible P waves. Although the QRS complexes and T waves are distinct, they certainly seem to be merging into a single configuration (note particularly lead aVR). Could this be some kind of idioventricular rhythm (see page 140)? Well, perhaps, but the clinical context argues for another interpretation. Both trimethoprim–methoxazole and lisinopril can cause hyperkalemia that is usually mild, but combined, they can cause severe, even life-threatening elevations in the serum potassium. And that's what you are seeing here—severe EKG manifestations of hyperkalemia, with a loss of P waves and broadened QRS complexes that are beginning to merge with the T waves to create a sine wave pattern.

Because of the risk of ventricular fibrillation in this setting, you send Ursula right to the emergency room where she is treated aggressively for hyperkalemia, taken off her medications, and monitored in the CCU until her EKG returns to normal. Eventually she is discharged on a different antibiotic and a different class of medication for her blood pressure. She does very well and declares that you are the best clinician she has ever met and will recommend you to all her new friends.

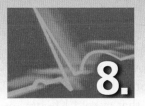

8. Putting It All Together

In this chapter you will learn:

1 | a simple method to incorporate everything you have learned into a step-by-step analysis of any EKG

2 | that all good things must come to an end, and we bid you a reluctant and fond farewell!

And that is really all there is to it.

Well, perhaps not quite all. What we need now is a way to organize all of this information, a simple methodical approach that can be applied to each and every EKG. It is important that every EKG be approached in an orderly fashion, particularly while you are still new at this, so that nothing important is missed. As you read more and more cardiograms, what initially may seem forced and mechanical will pay big dividends and will soon seem like second nature.

Two admonitions:

1. *Know your patient.* It is true that EKGs can be read with fair accuracy in a little back room in total isolation, but the power of this tool only really emerges when it is integrated into a total clinical assessment (*e.g.*, in Case 11 that we just concluded).

2. *Read EKGs.* Then read some more. Read them wherever you can find them—in books, in papers, in patients' charts, on bathroom walls. And read other books; this may be the only EKG book you will ever need, but it should not be the only one you will ever *want* to read. There are many outstanding textbooks, each with something special to offer.

There are as many approaches to reading EKGs as there are cardiologists. Everyone ultimately arrives at a method that works best for him or her. The following 11-Step Method is probably no better and no worse than most others. The first four steps are largely data gathering. The remainder are directed at specific diagnoses.

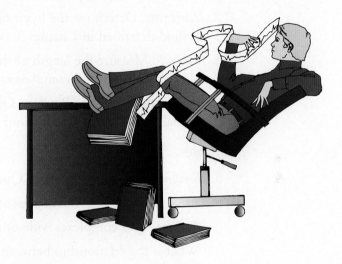

The 11-Step Method for Reading EKGs

Data Gathering

1. *Standardization.* Make sure the standardization mark on the EKG paper is 10 mm high so that 10 mm = 1 mV. Also make sure that the paper speed is correct.

2. *Heart rate.* Determine the heart rate by the quick three-step method described in Chapter 3.

3. *Intervals.* Measure the length of the PR and QT intervals and the width of the QRS complexes.

4. *Axis.* Is the axis of the P waves, QRS complexes, and T waves normal, or is there axis deviation?

Diagnoses

5. *Rhythm.* Always ask The Four Questions:

   Are there normal P waves present?

   Are the QRS complexes wide or narrow?

   What is the relationship between the P waves and QRS complexes?

   Is the rhythm regular or irregular?

6. *Atrioventricular (AV) block.* Apply the criteria in Chapter 4.

7. *Bundle branch block or hemiblock.* Apply the criteria in Chapter 4.

8. *Preexcitation.* Apply the criteria in Chapter 5.

(Note that steps 6 through 8 all involve looking for disturbances of conduction.)

9. *Enlargement and hypertrophy.* Apply the criteria for both atrial enlargement and ventricular hypertrophy.

10. *Coronary artery disease.* Look for Q waves and ST segment and T wave changes. Remember that not all such changes reflect coronary artery disease; know your differential diagnoses.

11. *Utter confusion.* Is there anything on the EKG you don't understand? Can it be explained by any of the noncardiac or unusual cardial conditions discussed in Chapter 7? Are you totally lost? Never hesitate to ask for assistance.

The following pages are memory joggers you can hang onto. Cut them out and stick them in that little black book of medical pearls that you carry around with you next to your smart phone. Cut them out anyway, even if you no longer carry a little black book; the exercise will do you good after sitting and staring bleary-eyed at this book for so long.

The final chapter contains some sample EKGs for you to test yourself with. Some are easy; some are not. But here is an interesting note: all of these patients were seen by one physician in a single day! This should give you an idea of how common EKG abnormalities can be and how important it is to be able to read the darn things.

And if you are still thinking, "Is this really all there is to it?," the answer—reminding you that information only becomes knowledge with wisdom and experience—is, "Yes!"

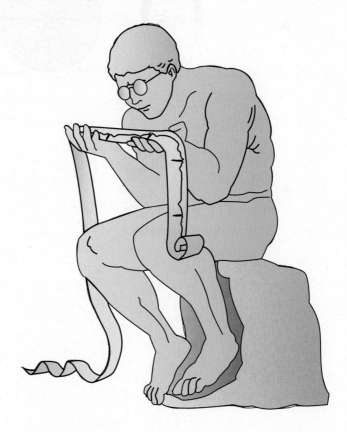

Review Charts

The 12 Leads

Anterior leads: V1, V2, V3, V4

Inferior leads: II, III, AVF

Left lateral leads: I, AVL, V5, V6

Right leads: aVR, V1

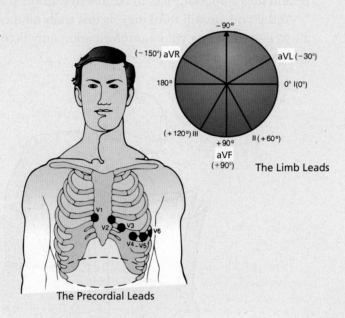

The Limb Leads

The Precordial Leads

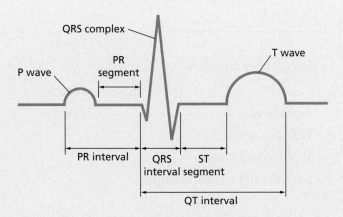

The heart is composed of pacemaker cells, electrical conducting cells, and myocardial cells. *Pacemaker* cells depolarize spontaneously and initiate each wave of depolarization. The SA node is usually the dominant pacemaker. *Electrical conducting cells* carry current rapidly and efficiently to distant regions of the heart. *Myocardial cells* constitute the bulk of the heart. When a wave of depolarization reaches a myocardial cell, calcium is released within the cell (excitation–contraction coupling), causing it to contract.

The P wave represents atrial depolarization. It is small and usually positive in the left lateral and inferior leads. It is often biphasic in leads III and V1. Typically, it is most positive in lead II and most negative in lead aVR.

The *QRS complex* represents ventricular depolarization. It is usually predominantly positive in most lateral and inferior leads. Across the precordium, the R waves increase in size, progressing from V1 to V5. A small initial Q wave, representing septal depolarization, can often be seen in the left lateral and inferior leads.

The *T wave* represents ventricular repolarization. It is the most variable waveform, but it is usually positive in leads with tall R waves.

The *PR interval* represents the time from the start of atrial depolarization to the start of ventricular depolarization.

The *PR segment* is the time from the end of atrial depolarization to the start of ventricular depolarization.

The *QRS interval* represents the duration of the QRS complex.

The *ST segment* represents the time from the end of ventricular depolarization to the start of ventricular repolarization.

The *QT interval* represents the time from the start of ventricular depolarization to the end of ventricular repolarization.

Calculating the Axis

	Lead I	Lead aVF
Normal axis	+	+
Left axis deviation	+	–
Right axis deviation	–	+
Extreme right axis deviation	–	–

Atrial Enlargement

Look at the P wave in leads II and V1.

Right atrial enlargement is characterized by the following:

1. Increased amplitude of the first portion of the P wave

2. No change in the duration of the P wave

3. Possible right axis deviation of the P wave.

Left atrial enlargement is characterized by the following:

1. Occasionally, increased amplitude of the terminal component of the P wave

2. More consistently, increased P wave duration

3. No significant axis deviation.

Ventricular Hypertrophy

Look at the QRS complexes in all leads.

Right ventricular hypertrophy is characterized by the following:

1. Right axis deviation of greater than 100°

2. Ratio of R wave amplitude to S wave amplitude greater than 1 in V1 and less than 1 in V6.

Left ventricular hypertrophy is characterized by many criteria. The more that are present, the greater the likelihood that left ventricular hypertrophy is present.

Precordial criteria include the following:

1. The R wave amplitude in V5 or V6 plus the S wave amplitude in V1 or V2 exceeds 35 mm.

2. The R wave amplitude in V5 exceeds 26 mm.

3. The R wave amplitude in V6 exceeds 18 mm.

4. The R wave amplitude in V6 exceeds the R wave amplitude in V5.

Limb lead criteria include the following:

1. The R wave amplitude in aVL exceeds 13 mm.

2. The R wave amplitude in aVF exceeds 21 mm.

3. The R wave amplitude in I exceeds 14 mm.

4. The R wave amplitude in I *plus* the S wave amplitude in III exceeds 25 mm.

The presence of repolarization abnormalities (asymmetric ST segment depression and T wave inversion) indicates clinically significant hypertrophy, is most often seen in those leads with tall R waves, and may herald ventricular dilatation and failure.

The four basic types of arrhythmias are as follows:

1. Arrhythmias of sinus origin

2. Ectopic rhythms

3. Conduction blocks

4. Preexcitation syndromes.

Whenever you are interpreting the heart's rhythm, ask The Four Questions:

1. Are normal P waves present?

2. Are the QRS complexes narrow (less than 0.12 seconds in duration) or wide (greater than 0.12 seconds)?

3. What is the relationship between the P waves and the QRS complexes?

4. Is the rhythm regular or irregular?

The answers for normal sinus rhythm are the following:

1. Yes, P waves are present.

2. The QRS complexes are narrow.

3. There is one P wave for every QRS complex.

4. The rhythm is regular.

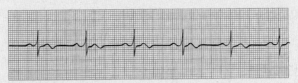

(A) Normal sinus rhythm.

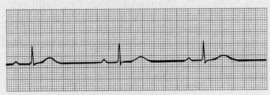

(B) Sinus tachycardia.

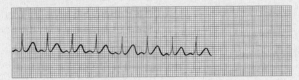

(C) Sinus bradycardia.

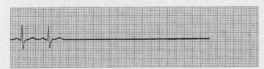

(D) Sinus arrest or exit block.

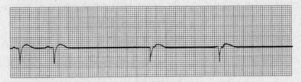

(E) Sinus arrest or exit block with junctional escape.

Supraventricular Arrhythmias

	Characteristics	EKG
Paroxysmal supraventricular tachycardia (PSVT)	Regular P waves are retrograde if visible Rate: 150 to 250 bpm Carotid massage: slows or terminates	
Flutter	Regular, saw-toothed 2:1, 3:1, 4:1, etc., block Atrial rate: 250 to 350 bpm Ventricular rate: one-half, one-third, one-fourth, etc., of the atrial rate Carotid massage: increases block	
Fibrillation	Irregular Undulating baseline Atrial rate: 350 to 500 bpm Ventricular rate: variable Carotid massage: may slow ventricular rate	
Multifocal atrial tachycardia *(MAT)*	Irregular At least three different P wave morphologies Rate: Usually 100 to 200 bpm; sometimes less than 100 bpm Carotid massage: no effect	
Paroxysmal atrial tachycardia *(PAT)*	Regular Rate: 100 to 200 bpm Characteristic warm-up period in the automatic form Carotid massage: no effect, or only mild slowing	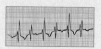

Ventricular Arrhythmias

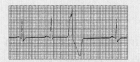

(A) Premature ventricular contractions (PVCs).

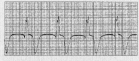

(D) Accelerated idioventricular rhythm.

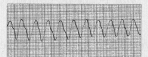

(B) Ventricular tachycardia.

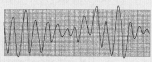

(E) Torsades de pointes.

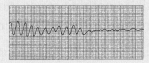

(C) Ventricular fibrillation.

Rules of Aberrancy

	Ventricular tachycardia (VT)	Paroxysmal supraventricular tachycardia (PSVT)
Clinical Clues		
Clinical history	Diseased heart	Usually normal heart
Carotid massage	No response	May terminate
Cannon A waves	May be present	Not seen
EKG Clues		
AV dissociation	May be seen	Not seen
Regularity	Slightly irregular	Very regular
Fusion beats	May be seen	Not seen
Initial QRS deflection	May differ from normal QRS complex	Same as normal QRS complex

AV Blocks

AV block is diagnosed by examining the relationship of the P waves to the QRS complexes.

1. *First degree*: The PR interval is greater than 0.2 second; all beats are conducted through to the ventricles.

2. *Second degree*: Only *some* beats are conducted through to the ventricles.

    a. *Mobitz type I (Wenckebach):* Progressive prolongation of the PR interval until a QRS is dropped

    b. *Mobitz type II*: All-or-nothing conduction in which QRS complexes are dropped without PR interval prolongation

3. *Third degree*: No beats are conducted through to the ventricles. There is complete heart block with AV dissociation in which the atria and ventricles are driven by independent pacemakers.

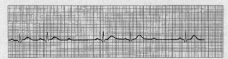

(A) First-degree AV block.   (B) Mobitz type I second-degree AV block (Wenckebach block).

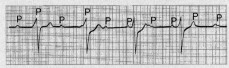

(C) Mobitz type II second-degree AV block.

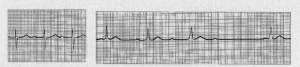

(D) Third-degree AV block.

Bundle Branch Blocks

Bundle branch block is diagnosed by looking at the width and configuration of the QRS complexes.

Criteria for Right Bundle Branch Block

1. QRS complex widened to greater than 0.12 seconds
2. RSR′ in leads V1 and V2 (rabbit ears) with ST segment depression and T wave inversion
3. Reciprocal changes in leads V5, V6, I, and aVL.

Criteria for Left Bundle Branch Block

1. QRS complex widened to greater than 0.12 seconds
2. Broad or notched R wave with prolonged upstroke in leads V5, V6, I, and aVL with ST segment depression and T wave inversion
3. Reciprocal changes in V1 and V2
4. Left axis deviation may be present.

Hemiblocks

Hemiblock is diagnosed by looking for left or right axis deviation.

Left Anterior Hemiblock

1. Normal QRS duration and no ST segment or T wave changes

2. Left axis deviation greater than −30°

3. No other cause of left axis deviation is present.

Left Posterior Hemiblock

1. Normal QRS duration and no ST segment or T wave changes

2. Right axis deviation

3. No other cause of right axis deviation is present.

Bifascicular Block

The features of the right bundle branch block combined with the left anterior hemiblock are as follows:

Right Bundle Branch Block

• QRS wider than 0.12 seconds

• RSR′ in V1 and V2.

Left Anterior Hemiblock

• Left axis deviation.

The features of the right bundle branch block combined with the left posterior hemiblock are as follows:

Right Bundle Branch Block

• RS wider than 0.12 seconds

• RSR′ in V1 and V2.

Left Posterior Hemiblock

- Right axis deviation.

Preexcitation

Criteria for Wolff-Parkinson-White (WPW) Syndrome

1. PR interval less than 0.12 seconds

2. Wide QRS complexes

3. Delta wave seen in some leads.

Criteria for Lown-Ganong-Levine (LGL) Syndrome

1. PR interval less than 0.12 seconds

2. Normal QRS width

3. No delta wave.

Arrhythmias commonly seen include the following:

1. Paroxysmal supraventricular tachycardia—narrow QRS complexes are more common than wide ones.

2. Atrial fibrillation—can be very rapid and can lead to ventricular fibrillation.

Myocardial Infarction

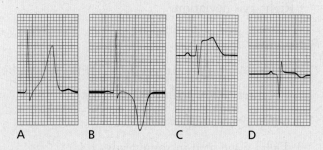

A   B   C   D

The diagnosis of a myocardial infarction is made by history, physical examination, serial cardiac enzyme determinations, and serial EKGs. During an acute infarction, the EKG evolves through three stages:

1. The T wave peaks (*A*) and then inverts (*B*).

2. The ST segment elevates (*C*).

3. Q waves appear (*D*).

Criteria for Significant Q Waves

1. The Q wave must be greater than 0.04 seconds in duration.

2. The depth of the Q wave must be at least one-third the height of the R wave in the same QRS complex.

Criteria for Non–Q Wave Infarctions

1. T wave inversion

2. ST segment depression persisting for more than 48 hours in the appropriate setting.

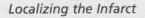

Localizing the Infarct

Inferior infarction: leads II, III, and aVF

Often caused by occlusion of the right coronary artery or its descending branch

Reciprocal changes in anterior and left lateral leads.

Lateral infarction: leads I, aVL, V5, and V6

Often caused by occlusion of the left circumflex artery

Reciprocal changes in inferior leads.

Anterior infarction: any of the precordial leads (V1 through V6)

Often caused by occlusion of the left anterior descending artery

Reciprocal changes in inferior leads

Posterior infarction: reciprocal changes in lead V1 (ST segment depression, tall R wave)

Often caused by occlusion of the right coronary artery.

The ST Segment

ST segment *elevation* may be seen

1. with an evolving infarction

2. in Prinzmetal's angina.

ST segment *depression* may be seen

1. with typical exertional angina

2. in a non–Q wave infarction.

ST *depression* is also one indicator of a positive stress test.

Other causes of ST segment *elevation:*

J point elevation

Apical ballooning syndrome

Acute pericarditis

Acute myocarditis

Hyperkalemia

Pulmonary embolism

Brugada syndrome

Hypothermia

Miscellaneous EKG Changes

Electrolyte Disturbances

- *Hyperkalemia:* Evolution of peaked T waves, PR prolongation and P wave flattening, and QRS widening. Ultimately, the QRS complexes and T waves merge to form a sine wave, and ventricular fibrillation may develop.

- *Hypokalemia:* ST depression, T wave flattening, U waves

- *Hypocalcemia:* Prolonged QT interval

- *Hypercalcemia:* Shortened QT interval.

Hypothermia

- Osborn waves, prolonged intervals, sinus bradycardia, slow atrial fibrillation; beware of muscle tremor artifact.

Drugs

- *Digitalis:* Therapeutic levels associated with ST segment and T wave changes in leads with tall R waves; toxic levels associated with tachyarrhythmias and conduction blocks; PAT with block is most characteristic.

- *Sotalol, quinidine, procainamide, disopyramide, amiodarone, dofetilide, dronedarone, tricyclic antidepressants, erythromycin, the quinolones, the phenothiazines, various antifungal medications, some antihistamines:* prolonged QT interval, U waves.

Other Cardiac Disorders

- *Pericarditis:* Diffuse ST segment and T wave changes. A large effusion can cause low voltage and electrical alternans.

- *Hypertrophic cardiomyopathy*: Ventricular hypertrophy, left axis deviation, septal Q waves

- *Myocarditis:* Conduction blocks.

Pulmonary Disorders

- *Chronic obstructive pulmonary disease (COPD):* Low voltage, right axis deviation, poor R wave progression. Chronic cor pulmonale can produce P pulmonale and right ventricular hypertrophy with repolarization abnormalities.

- *Acute pulmonary embolism:* Right ventricular hypertrophy with strain, right bundle branch block, S1Q3. Sinus tachycardia and atrial fibrillation are the most common arrhythmias.

Central Nervous System Disease

- Diffuse T wave inversion, with T waves typically wide and deep; U waves.

The Athlete's Heart

- Sinus bradycardia, nonspecific ST segment and T wave changes, left and right ventricular hypertrophy, incomplete right bundle branch block, first-degree or Wenckebach AV block, occasional supraventricular arrhythmia.

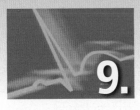

9. How Do You Get to Carnegie Hall?[1]

The following EKGs will allow you to try out your new skills. Use the 11-Step Method; don't overlook anything; take your time. Ready? Here we go:

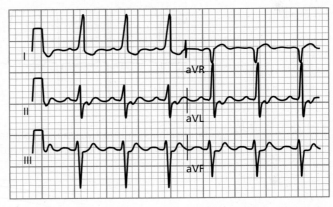

Sinus tachycardia. Note also the presence of left axis deviation.

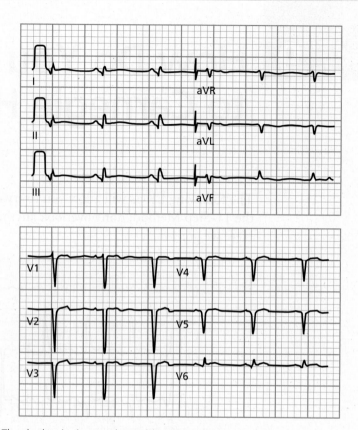

The rhythm is sinus tachycardia. Deep anterior Q waves and lateral Q waves indicate an anterolateral myocardial infarction.

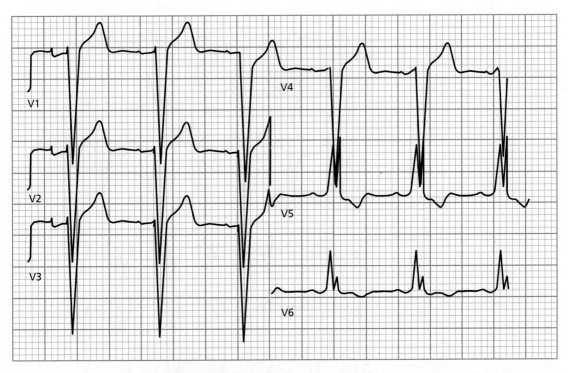

The QRS complexes are wide and distorted. In leads V5 and V6, the QRS complexes are notched, and there is ST segment depression and T wave inversion. This patient has left bundle branch block.

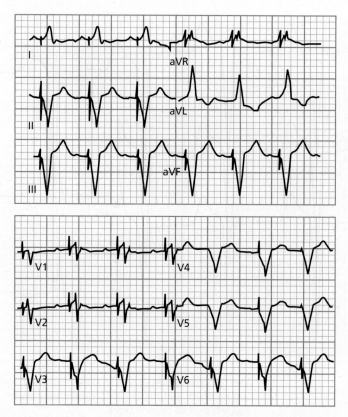

The broad, abnormal QRS complexes may immediately attract your attention, but notice the pacer spikes before each one. The spikes are preceded by a P wave (look at leads II, III, aVF, V1, and V2). This pacemaker fires whenever it senses a P wave, ensuring ventricular contraction.

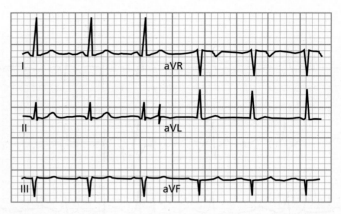

Note the deep Q waves in leads III and aVF. This tracing shows an inferior infarct.

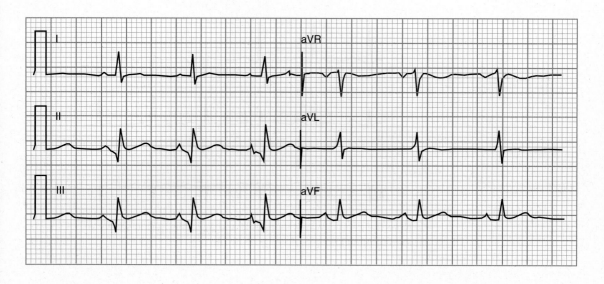

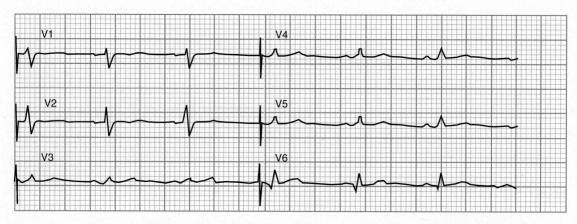

The salient features here are the short PR interval, the broadened QRS complex, and the telltale delta waves (best seen in leads aVL and aVF) of Wolff-Parkinson-White syndrome.

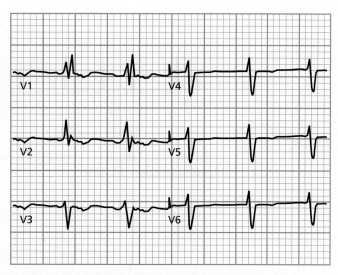

The QRS complexes are greatly widened, with beautiful rabbit ears in lead V1. This patient has right bundle branch block.

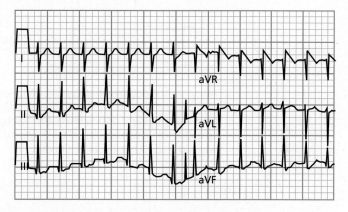

The rate is very fast and regular, and the QRS complexes are narrow. Retrograde P waves can be seen in lead III. This patient has a paroxysmal supraventricular tachycardia.

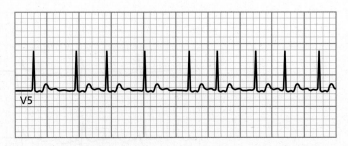

The rhythm is irregular, and the QRS complexes are narrow. This patient is in atrial fibrillation.

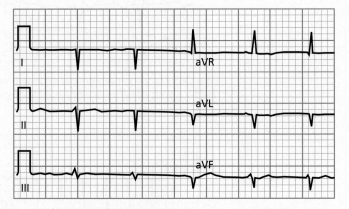

Are you confused by what appears to be extreme right axis deviation? Actually, in this instance, the EKG electrodes were accidentally reversed—the right arm and left arm electrodes were placed on the wrong arms. When you see a tall R wave in lead aVR and a deep S wave in lead I, check your electrodes.

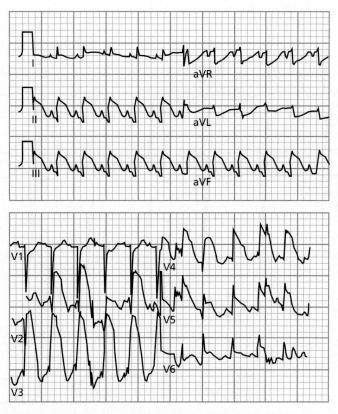

Everywhere you look, you see dramatic ST segment elevation. This EKG shows an evolving infarct affecting the entire heart!

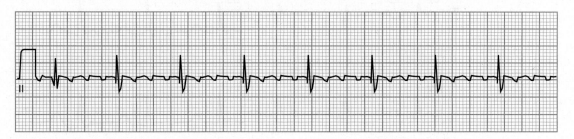

You are staring at the classic saw-toothed pattern of atrial flutter.

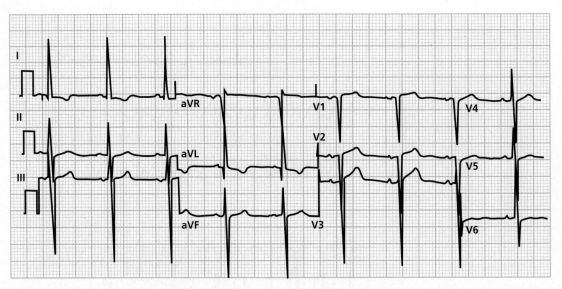

Left ventricular hypertrophy by all criteria.

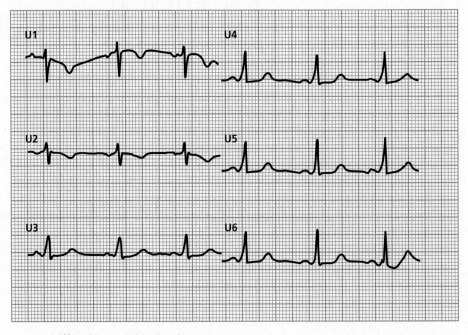

Wolff-Parkinson-White syndrome.

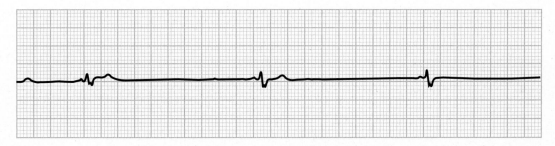

Extreme bradycardia resulting from hypoxemia in a patient with sleep apnea.

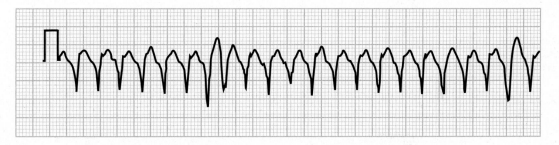

Atrial fibrillation with a rapid ventricular response.

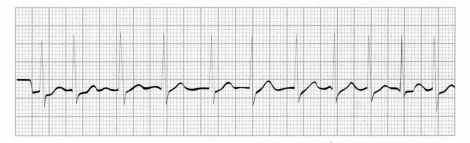

Ventricular tachycardia.

Index

Note: Page numbers followed by *f* indicate figures.